W9-BID-932

Pediatric
and Adolescent
Gynecology

PEDIATRIC AND ADOLESCENT GYNECOLOGY

S. JEAN HERRIOT EMANS, M.D.
Instructor in Pediatrics, Harvard Medical School;
Associate Chief, Division of Adolescent Medicine,
The Children's Hospital Medical Center, Boston

DONALD PETER GOLDSTEIN, M.D.
Assistant Clinical Professor in Obstetrics
and Gynecology, Harvard Medical School;
Chief, Division of Gynecology,
The Children's Hospital Medical Center, Boston

LITTLE, BROWN AND COMPANY   BOSTON

Copyright © 1977 by Little, Brown and Company (Inc.)

First Edition

All rights reserved. No part of this book may be reproduced in any form or by any electronic or mechanical means, including information storage and retrieval systems, without permission in writing from the publisher, except by a reviewer who may quote brief passages in a review.

Library of Congress Catalog Card No. 76-46865

ISBN 0-316-23400-1

Printed in the United States of America

TO OUR FAMILIES

Preface

Over the past few years many pediatricians, family practitioners, and nurses have expressed an interest in a simplified approach to the common gynecological problems of the child and the adolescent. Problems such as the differential diagnosis of ambiguous genitalia, vulvovaginitis, and precocious development arise in the care of infants and children. Dysmenorrhea, irregular periods, venereal disease, and pregnancy represent common presenting complaints of the adolescent. Perhaps because of the fear of not knowing enough or possible trauma to the young patient, family physicians have often referred all girls with minor problems directly to the gynecologist. In fact, a little girl is often more comfortable seeing her own familiar doctor, and the adolescent benefits greatly from the unhurried approach of the generalist; the statement "Your pelvic examination is normal" answers few questions.

Many gynecological problems can be diagnosed on the basis of the general physical examination, including rectal-abdominal palpation; it is hoped that many practitioners will feel comfortable doing a vaginal examination as well. A step-by-step description of the routine examination of the child and adolescent is given in Chapter 1. In Chapter 4 the physiology of puberty is briefly reviewed as a background to the common menstrual problems of the adolescent. Mastery of these two chapters is essential before proceeding to the diagnosis and treatment of gynecological problems.

Practicing physicians can often gain additional experience by working with a local gynecologist in his office or in a family planning clinic. It is hoped that in the future house officers will become reasonably proficient as medical gynecologists during their training years. In a similar fashion, the nurse and nurse-practitioner should find this book a handy reference.

In general, discussion is focused on the most common diagnoses rather than on rare conditions that the generalist is unlikely to see in his lifetime. Additional references are listed at the end of many chapters for the physician or nurse interested in more in-depth reading on a particular problem. Treatment regimens included in each section are intended as suggestions, not as the only method of therapy. We have also tried to include a brief discussion of some of the major psychological issues involved in pregnancy, rape, and sexuality counseling. Some problems will clearly require referral to a gynecologist; ideally, a sympathetic physician interested in children and adolescents can be chosen.

As authors, we hope to stimulate the physician to become more proficient and knowledgeable in the medical-gynecological care of the child and the adolescent. Working together for the past two years, we have tried to establish a comprehensive program for gynecological service and teaching, utilizing two nurse counselors in the Gynecology Clinic and a nurse practitioner and Fellows in the Adolescents' Unit. This book represents an approach that we have found successful at the Children's Hospital Medical Center, Boston.

We thank the many people who helped in the preparation of the book, including John F. Crigler, Jr., M.D., Arnold Smith, M.D., and Diane Kittredge, M.D., all of whom reviewed chapters of the book; Dr. Robert P. Masland, Jr., for his many helpful suggestions and his authorship of the chapter on sex education; Miss Patricia Coiffi, Mrs. Ruth Mersereau, and Miss Catherine Lydon for technical assistance; Miss Laurette Langlois for her many artistic contributions; and most especially Mrs. Peggy Webb, who typed the entire manuscript in record time.

S. J. H. E.
D. P. G.

Boston

Contents

Pediatric
and Adolescent
Gynecology

NOTICE

The indications and dosages of all drugs in this book have been recommended in the medical literature and conform to the practices of the general medical community. The medications described do not necessarily have specific approval by the Food and Drug Administration for use in the diseases and dosages for which they are recommended in this book. The package insert for each drug should be consulted for use and dosage as approved by the F.D.A. Because standards for usage change, it is advisable to keep abreast of revised recommendations, particularly those concerning new drugs.

1. Office Evaluation of the Child and Adolescent

OFFICE EVALUATION OF THE INFANT AND CHILD

The traditional Victorian avoidance of the female external genitalia has unfortunately often prevented mothers and physicians from dealing with the total health care of the young girl. Although gynecological problems are not common among young girls, the physician should always include inspection of the external genitalia and breast palpation as part of the routine physical examination. If the child accepts a brief look at her genitalia as part of the normal physical, she is less likely to feel embarrassed or upset by the same examination when she reaches adolescence. In addition, the physician may note smegma or feces in the labial folds, indicating inadequate perineal hygiene. Careful instruction to the mother and child at that time may prevent the later occurrence of a nonspecific vulvovaginitis. A cyst, clitoromegaly, early signs of puberty, or monilial vulvitis may be a clue to another problem. Errors in diagnosis often stem from lack of simple inspection.

Obtaining the History

Discharge, vaginal bleeding, pruritus, or signs of sexual development should prompt a more thorough evaluation. The history obviously depends on the presenting complaint. If the problem is vaginitis, questions should focus on perineal hygiene, antibiotic therapy, and recent infections in the patient or other members of the family. *Trichomonas*, group A β-hemolytic *Streptococcus*, gonorrhea, and condyloma acuminata may be spread by close (not necessarily sexual) contact. If the problem is vaginal bleeding, the history should include recent growth and development, signs of puberty, use of hormone creams or tablets, and a previous finding of foreign bodies in the vagina. In all patients, regardless of the symptoms, a history of in utero exposure to diethylstilbestrol (DES) should be recorded. Routine gynecological examination is not indicated in the asymptomatic prepubertal child because clear cell adenocarcinoma of the vagina has been reported only rarely before menarche; however, *any* complaint of discharge or bleeding should receive prompt attention. The implications of DES and the routine examination of the postmenarcheal adolescent are discussed in detail in Chapter 10. Although the history is usually obtained chiefly from the mother (and sometimes the father), the older child should certainly be given a few moments alone with the physician to ask her own questions. This time promotes an understanding that the physician is acting in her best interests.

GYNECOLOGICAL EXAMINATION

The gynecological examination should be carefully explained in advance to the mother and the child. It is extremely important to tell the mother that the size of the vaginal opening is quite variable and that the exam will in no way alter the hymen. Often a diagram showing the introitus is helpful because many mothers still believe that the virginal introitus is totally covered by the hymen (Fig. 1-1).

An aura of mystery often surrounds the exam of the virginal girl, especially if she is prepubertal. Both mother and child should be told that instruments will be used that are specially designed for little girls. If an eyedropper or Q-Tip is to be used, the child should have a chance to feel it. The nurse should then instruct the child to empty her bladder and undress. Whether or not the mother should stay in the room depends on the physician's assessment of the child and the

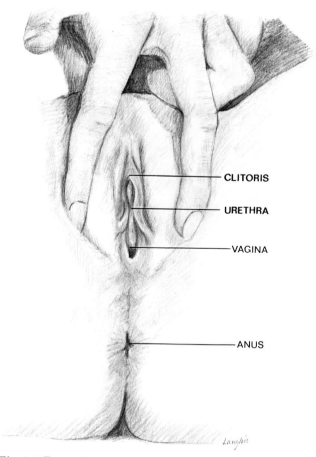

Fig. 1-1. External genitalia of the prepubertal girl.

mother. Little girls are usually most comfortable in the mother's lap or holding her hand; older girls usually prefer to be examined in stirrups with the mother out of the room. If the physician is confident and relaxed, the patient usually responds with cooperation. An abrupt or hurried approach will precipitate anxiety and resistance in the child.

The examination of any patient having gynecological complaints should include a general pediatric assessment of the child's nutrition, head and neck, heart, lungs, and abdomen. The abdominal exam is often easier if the child places her hand on the examiner's hand; she is then less apt to tense her muscles or complain of being "tickled." The inguinal areas should be carefully palpated for a hernia or gonad; occasionally the inguinal gonad is the testis of an undiagnosed male pseudohermaphrodite. The breasts should be carefully inspected and palpated. Increasing diameter of the areola or a unilateral tender breast bud is often the first sign of puberty.

The gynecological exam of the child includes inspection of the external genitalia, visualization of the vagina and cervix, and rectal-abdominal palpation. This exam is usually possible without anesthesia if the child has not been traumatized by previous exams and if the physician proceeds slowly. The child should be explicitly told that "the exam will not hurt." The young child should be on her back with her knees apart and feet touching; the older child can be examined with the use of adjustable stirrups. As the external genitalia are inspected, the young child is usually less anxious if she assists the physician by holding the labia apart. The physician should note the presence of pubic hair, clitoral size, signs of estrogenization of the vaginal introitus, and perineal hygiene. The size of the clitoral glans in the premenarcheal child should not exceed 3 mm in length and 2 mm in transverse diameter [1]. The vaginal mucosa of the prepubertal child appears thin and red in contrast to the moist, dull pink, estrogenized mucosa of the pubertal child. The vaginal introitus often gaps open if the child is asked to take a deep breath or cough. If not, the labia should be gently pulled downward and laterally. Occasionally a saline-moistened Q-Tip or urethral catheter is necessary to check for vaginal patency. If a cystic hymenal or vaginal tag is found, excision may be in order to rule out the highly malignant sarcoma botryoides. The anus and labia should always be examined for cleanliness, excoriations, and erythema. Perianal excoriation is often a clue to the presence of a pinworm infestation.

Once the external genitalia have been carefully examined, the physician should proceed with visualization of the vagina. In girls over 2 years old, the knee-chest position provides a particularly good view of the vagina and cervix without instrumentation. The patient is told that she should "lie on her tummy with her bottom in the air." She is reassured that the examiner plans to "take a look at her bottom" but "will not put anything inside her." In the knee-chest position (also used for sigmoidoscopy in older patients), the child rests her head to one side on her folded arms and supports her remaining weight on bended knees (6 to 8 inches apart). With her buttocks held up in the air, she is encouraged to let her spine and stomach "sag downward." An assistant helps to hold the buttocks apart, pressing laterally and slightly upward. As the child takes deep breaths, the vaginal orifice falls open for examination (Fig. 1-2). An ordinary otoscope head (without a speculum) provides the magnification and light necessary to visualize the cervix. Clearly the child's anxiety will be allayed if she is shown the otoscope light and her full confidence is gained before this part of the exam. A running conversation of small talk about school, toys, and siblings often diverts the child's attention and helps her to maintain this position for several minutes without moving or objecting. Since the vagina of the prepubertal child is quite short, the presence of a foreign body or a lesion is often easily ascertained.

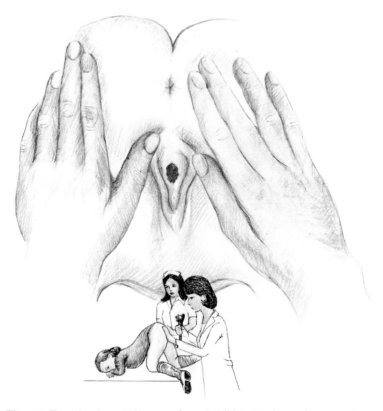

Fig. 1-2. Examination of the prepubertal child in the knee-chest position.

An alternate method of visualization is the use of a small vagino-scope or cystoscope. The child is examined supine with her knees held apart. An excellent step-by-step method of inserting the vaginoscope in the young child has been introduced by Dr. Capraro of Buffalo [2]. The child is first allowed to touch the instrument and told that it feels "slippery, funny, and cool." The instrument is then placed against her inner thigh and the same words are repeated. Next the instrument is placed against her labia, again with the words "This feels slippery, funny, and cool." As the vaginoscope is inserted through the hymen, the examiner repeats the words and presses the child's buttocks firmly with his other hand to divert her attention. Good visualization of the cervix and vagina is thus possible without anes-thesia. Since it is unlikely that the general physician will have a vaginoscope or cystoscope in the office, several plastic specula have been designed to fit on the standard pediatric otoscope. In addition, a vaginal speculum ($3 \times 5\!/\!8$ inches) can be used in the older child if insertion does not cause excessive pain and trauma.

If a vaginal discharge is present, samples should be obtained for culture, Gram's stain, and wet and potassium hydroxide (KOH) preparations (see p. 16). If a tumor is suspected, a smear should be sent for cytology. Usually the child prefers to lie on her back with her knees apart so that she can watch the procedure without becoming excessively anxious. If only one sample is necessary, a saline-moistened cotton-tipped applicator can be inserted into the vagina. If several samples are necessary, a soft plastic eyedropper (such as a Clinitest* dropper) or a glass eyedropper with 4–5 cm of intravenous plastic tubing attached [3] can be gently inserted through the hymen to aspirate secretions. The patient should be allowed to touch an appli-cator or eyedropper before it is actually inserted and told, "This is soft. Feel it; it won't hurt you." Since quite small quantities of the discharge are often obtained, a tube of Brain Heart Infusion (BHI)† broth can be inoculated with one small drop. If the discharge is copious and purulent, cultures should be planted on blood, McConkey's, and Thayer-Martin (or Transgrow†) media.

After the samples are obtained, a gentle rectal-abdominal examina-tion is done, with the patient in stirrups or supine with her legs apart. The examiner places the index or fifth finger of one hand into the rectum and the other hand on the abdomen for bimanual palpation. Since the child has usually previously experienced the sensation of a rectal thermometer, she can be reassured that this exam will feel the same to her. Except in the newborn period when the uterus is enlarged secondary to maternal estrogen, the rectal exam in the prepubertal

---

* Ames Co., Division of Miles Laboratories, Elkhart, Ind. 46514.
† Scott Laboratories, Fiskeville, R.I. 02823.

child reveals only the small "button" of the cervix. Since the ovaries are not palpable, adnexal masses should alert the physician to the possibility of a cyst or tumor.

After assessing the presenting complaint and the results of the examination, the physician should spend time with the mother and child discussing the diagnosis, mode of therapy, and necessity of follow-up. Praising the young child for her cooperation and "bravery" helps to establish the important doctor-patient relationship for future exams.

OFFICE EVALUATION OF THE ADOLESCENT

The evaluation of the adolescent requires additional technical skills, including speculum examination of the vagina and rectal-vaginal-abdominal palpation. More importantly, the physician needs the interpersonal skills, sensitivity, and time to establish a primary relationship with the adolescent herself. The doctor must be willing to see the teenager alone and listen to her concerns. For example, the patient with oligomenorrhea may return each visit with the same question: "Why am I not normal?" Listening to her describe her feelings is just as important as drawing diagrams of the hypothalamic-ovarian axis. The statement "Your pelvic exam is normal" answers few questions for the adolescent.

Indeed, imagining the body changes involved in the development of the prepubertal latency-age girl of 10 into the sexually mature woman of 20 underscores the many issues that arise in the medical care of adolescent girls. Pubic hair and breast development, over which the girl has no control, can be quite distressing. The fact that these changes occur at the same rate as her peer group may offer some reassurance; to be early or late can provoke considerable anxiety. A 12-year-old girl who looks 16 may be confronted with heterosexual demands that she is unable to cope with; a 16-year-old girl who looks 10 may be embarrassed to undress in physical education class or to interact with her peer group. Since the young adolescent has many fantasies about her body and its changes, she may ask the same questions at each visit. The older teenager of 16 or 17 years of age is better equipped to deal with the diagnosis on an intellectual level. The physician must, therefore, be sensitive to the different needs of each patient.

Obtaining the History

The source of the medical history depends on the setting and the age of the patient. The older adolescent tends to seek gynecological care on her own initiative. In a clinic setting, the mother (and father) may be seen by the physician first to ascertain the nature of the chief complaint, as well as the past medical history, school problems, and psychosocial adjustment. Most of the visit should be devoted to seeing the teenager alone, since often her presenting complaint is quite different from her mother's concerns. In private practice, the mother may make the appointment by telephone and then the teenager may appear alone for the examination.

The history sheet shown in Figure 1-3 is currently used in our gynecology clinic. As it indicates, the general medical history is quite relevant in the evaluation of gynecological problems. The routine visit with the adolescent should always include a carefully taken menstrual history and a straightforward question about sexual relations and birth control. The physician's guarantee of confidentiality should be explicitly stated, because few teenagers will volunteer a need for birth control. A useful question may be, "If you make a decision to have sexual relations, would you know how to protect yourself from pregnancy?" Or "If you had a girl friend who didn't want to get pregnant, could you help her?" If she says yes, ask "How?" Such discussions require skillful handling, since repeatedly offering birth control advice may push a young woman into premature sexual relations that she may regret. Frequently pointing out that 50 percent of adolescents have not had intercourse by their nineteenth birthday reassures the patient who would like to remain virginal but believes that all her friends are sexually active.

It is not uncommon to find that a 13- or 14-year-old girl with school problems, mother-daughter conflict, and a history of running away is involved in unprotected intercourse as part of her so-called acting out. Intercourse is rarely associated in the adolescent mind with pregnancy and motherhood. The older teenager of 16 or 17 years of age is more likely to consider the consequences of her actions, but nevertheless she too may fail to obtain birth control. The physician may feel in an ethical bind: To push birth control implies approval; to deny birth control may result in an unwanted pregnancy. Although the physician may have strong opinions regarding the morality of premarital intercourse, defining the issues under discussion is more helpful than a stilted, pedantic lecture. Identifying alternatives may direct the adolescent to an acceptable solution. Concerned medical care that is sensitive to her needs will hopefully assist her in the development of a healthy body image and responsible sexuality.

GYNECOLOGICAL EXAMINATION

Once the history is obtained and the problems identified, the patient should be given a gown and asked to remove all her clothes including brassiere and underpants. If she is well draped and approached in a relaxed manner, resistance is unlikely. A female nurse (not the mother) in the room is often reassuring. The general physical exam of a teenage girl should always include a breast exam, inspection of

S. Jean Emans, M.D.

USE PLATE
OR PRINT

M R No _____ DATE _____

PT NAME _____

PARENT _____

ADDRESS _____

_____

DATE OF BIRTH _____ B C No _____

M A No _____

DIV _____ CLIN _____ P P DR _____

GYNECOLOGICAL HISTORY SHEET

THE CHILDREN'S HOSPITAL MEDICAL CENTER, BOSTON, MASSACHUSETTS 02115

REFERRED BY: _____ AGE: _____

MENSTRUAL HISTORY

MENARCHE _____

CYCLE _____ DURATION _____ AMT. _____

DYSMENORRHEA _____

INTERMENSTRUAL BLEEDING _____

LMP _____ PMP _____ WKS LMP _____

GYNECOLOGIC HISTORY

LAST PELVIC _____

LAST PAP _____

PREGNANCY TEST _____ RESULTS _____

DYSPAREUNIA _____

POST-COITAL BLEEDING _____

VAGINAL DISCHARGE _____

V.D. _____

MATERNAL·STILBESTROL _____

OBSTETRIC HISTORY

GRAVIDA _____ PARA _____

INDUCED ABS. _____ SPONT. ABS. _____

NO. OF LIVING CHILDREN _____

DATE OF LAST DELIVERY _____

NORMAL _____ C-SECT. _____

CONTRACEPTIVE HISTORY

TYPE _____

DURATION _____

PROBLEMS _____

_____

MEDICAL HISTORY

ANEMIA _____

HEART DISEASE _____

LUNG DISEASE _____

LIVER DISEASE _____

KIDNEY DISEASE _____

HYPERTENSION _____

MIGRAINE HEADACHES _____

THROMBOPHLEBITIS _____

EPILEPSY _____

DIABETES _____

ASTHMA _____

BREAST DISEASE _____

CANCER _____

PSYCHIATRIC CARE _____

SICKLE CELL _____

ALLERGIES _____

CURRENT MEDS. _____

HOSPITALIZATIONS _____

_____

SERIOUS ILLNESSES _____

_____

MAY WE CONTACT YOU AT HOME? ☐YES ☐NO

IF NOT, WHERE? _____

_____

16421 01 5C 6-74

Fig. 1-3. Gynecological history sheet.

the genitalia, and a careful notation of the Tanner stages of breast and pubic hair development (Chap. 4). Demonstrating self-examination of the breast to the patient as one actually performs the breast exam (Chap. 12) often puts the young woman at ease. Physicians and patients occasionally ask why it is necessary to look at the genitalia. There are a number of reasons: Monilial vulvitis may be the first sign of diabetes; an imperforate hymen may be the etiology of abdominal pain or primary amenorrhea; a cyst or clitoromegaly may be unexpectedly found. Not infrequently the actual exam initiates questions from the teenager that she was embarrassed to ask about, such as a vaginal discharge, a lump, or irregular periods.

When is a pelvic exam indicated? A bimanual rectal-abdominal exam (in the lithotomy position) should be performed on any teenager with gynecological complaints or unexplained abdominal pain. A vaginal exam is important for irregular bleeding, severe dysmenorrhea, discharge, in utero exposure to DES, venereal disease, and primary amenorrhea. Sexually active patients should have a routine vaginal examination every 6 to 12 months; patients who are not sexually active should begin routine annual examinations at the age of 17 or 18. Contrary to popular belief, rarely is a patient unable to be fully cooperative during a pelvic exam if she has received a careful explanation about the procedure and its importance in evaluating her individual problem.

The pelvic exam is done in the lithotomy position with the use of stirrups. The external genitalia are inspected first; estrogenization of the vaginal mucosa, distribution of the pubic hair, and the size of the clitoris are assessed. The estrogenized vagina has a succulent, dull pink mucosa in contrast to the thin, red mucosa of the prepubertal child. The normal clitoral glans is 2 to 4 mm in width; a width of 10 mm is considered significant virilization. The normal anatomy is illustrated in Figure 1-4. The variation in hymens found in the adolescent girl is shown in Figure 1-5. A simple hymenotomy is required prior to menarche for type B (imperforate hymen) and prior to intercourse in types C, D, and E. It is important that the adolescent with type C, D, or E hymen be aware of her anatomy and her inability to use tampons or have intercourse at that time. The timing of the hymenotomy should be the joint decision of the physician and the patient; the doctor should not arbitrarily tell the adolescent to wait until marriage.

To avoid surprising the patient, a manual or speculum examination should be preceded by a statement such as, "I'm now going to touch your bottom," or "I'm now going to place this cool metal speculum in your vagina." In the virginal teenager, a slow one-finger exam will demonstrate the size of the introitus and the location of the cervix to allow subsequent easy insertion of the speculum. It is helpful to warm the speculum and then touch it to the patient's thigh to allow

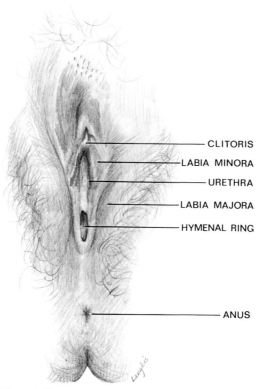

CLITORIS

LABIA MINORA

URETHRA

LABIA MAJORA

HYMENAL RING

ANUS

Fig. 1-4. External genitalia of the pubertal female.

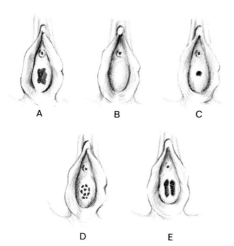

A   B   C

D   E

Fig. 1-5. Types of hymen: (A) *normal,* (B) *imperforate,* (C) *punctate,* (D) *cribriform,* (E) *septate.*

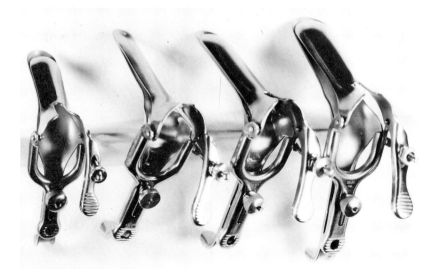

Fig. 1-6. Types of specula: infant, Huffman, Pederson, Graves (from left to right).

her to feel its "cool metal" quality. If the hymenal opening is small, a Huffman speculum (½ × 4¼ inches) is used to expose the cervix. In the sexually active teenager, a Pederson (1 × 4½ inches) or Graves (1⅜ × 3¾ inches) speculum is appropriate. A child's speculum (⅝ × 3 inches or ⅞ × 3 inches) is less useful because of inadequate length (Figs. 1-6 and 1-7). The stratified squamous epithelium of the cervix is usually a homogeneous dull pink color; however, in many adolescents an erythematous area surrounding the os is noted. This so-called congenital erosion is the presence of endocervical columnar epithelium on the cervix. The squamocolumnar junction, instead of being inside the endocervical canal, is visible on the portio of the cervix. Samples for the Papanicolaou smear, cultures, and wet and KOH preparations are taken with the speculum in place; the techniques are described in the section on diagnostic tests. After visualization of the vagina and cervix, the speculum is removed, and the uterus and adnexa are carefully palpated with one or two fingers in the vagina and the other hand on the abdomen (Fig. 1-8).

A rectal-vaginal-abdominal exam performed with the index finger in the vagina, the middle finger in the rectum, and the other hand on the abdomen permits palpation of a retroverted uterus and assessment of mobility of the adnexa and uterus. The patient is usually less anxious if she is told in advance that the rectal exam may seem disturbing because she will feel that she is "having a bowel movement on the table." Allaying this fear usually elicits better relaxation and cooperation (Fig. 1-9).

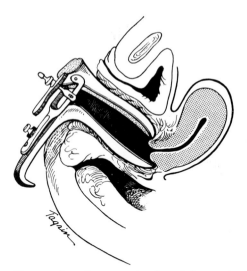

Fig. 1-7. Speculum examination of the cervix. (From T. Green [4]. Copyright, 1971, Little, Brown and Company, by permission.)

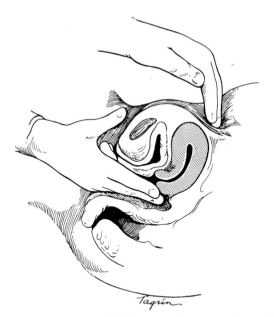

Fig. 1-8. Bimanual abdominovaginal palpation of the uterus. (From T. Green [4]. Copyright, 1971, Little, Brown and Company, by permission.)

13

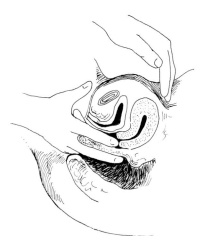

Fig. 1-9. Bidigital rectovaginal examination. (Adapted from T. Green [4]. Copyright, 1971, Little, Brown and Company, by permission.)

A simple bimanual rectal-abdominal examination with the index finger pushing the cervix upward allows palpation of the uterus and adnexa. In a relaxed patient, a negative exam rules out large ovarian masses and uterine enlargement.

After the examination is concluded and the patient has dressed, the physician should sit down and discuss the presenting complaint and findings in detail. It is essential that the adolescent be treated as an adult capable of understanding the explanation. If her mother has accompanied her, the patient should be asked whether she would like to tell her mother the findings herself or whether she would prefer to have the physician discuss the diagnosis in her presence. It is extremely important for the patient to know that the doctor and her mother will not have a "secret" about her and that confidential information will not be divulged to her mother.

DIAGNOSTIC TESTS
PAPANICOLAOU SMEAR
A Papanicolaou (Pap) smear should be taken on all young women who have a speculum examination. Although infrequent, cervical dysplasia and carcinoma do occur in teenagers. With the speculum in place, an Ayer wooden spatula is scraped around the cervix with a circular motion and the collected material is spread on a slide. In addition, a cotton-tipped applicator, moistened with saline, may then be inserted into the endocervical canal approximately 1/4 inch and twirled. The applicator is streaked across the same slide, and the slide is then placed in a bottle filled with Pap solution. The cytology laboratory returns a reading of class I, II, IIR, III, IV, or V as follows:

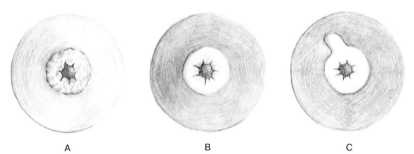

Fig. 1-10. Schiller's test: (A) congenital erosion, (B) normal Schiller's stain, (C) abnormal Schiller's stain. (Adapted from T. Green [4]. Copyright, 1971, Little, Brown and Company, by permission.)

   I. Negative
  II. Benign atypia (also considered negative)
IIR. Atypical cells
 III. Dysplasia
 IV. Suspicious for tumor cells, probably carcinoma in situ
  V. Definite tumor cells

Patients with class I or II smears are followed with annual Pap smears. Patients with class IIR smears usually have atypical cells secondary to a *Trichomonas* or *Candida* vaginitis, or endometrial cells are evident because the Pap smear was taken at the end of a menstrual period. Such patients should receive medication for the vaginitis and a repeat Pap smear in two to three months at midcycle. Patients with class III, IV, or V smears should be referred to a gynecologist for further evaluation and treatment. Schiller's iodine stain allows the gynecologist to take appropriate biopsies. The squamous cervical and vaginal epithelial cells take up the stain, producing a brown color, whereas the columnar epithelium of the endocervix and abnormal areas (carcinoma in situ, squamous metaplasia) do not take up the stain (Fig. 1-10). If the biopsies and Pap smear confirm the presence of dysplasia (class III), cryocauterization is indicated.

Vaginal Smear for Estrogen

In the absence of inflammation, a vaginal smear is useful for evaluating the patient's hormonal status. This smear is best obtained with the speculum in place by scraping the side wall of the vagina with a wooden tongue depressor or Q-Tip moistened with saline. However, the smear can be obtained without a speculum by inserting a moistened Q-Tip into the vaginal introitus. The cells obtained are streaked on a glass slide, and the slide is placed immediately in Pap fixative. The cytologist reads the smear by the number of parabasal, intermediate, and superficial cells. The greater the estrogen effect, the more superficial cells there are. The patient with little or no estrogen, such as the prepubertal child or the adolescent with amenorrhea secondary to anorexia nervosa, will have predominantly parabasal cells.

Percentage of Superficial Cells

Less than 5%	Poor estrogen effect
5–10%	Slight estrogen effect
10–30%	Moderate estrogen effect
Greater than 30%	Marked estrogen effect

The smear can be correlated with the clinical situation (Table 1-1).
Since the epithelial cells in the urine show the same hormonal changes, the urine of a prepubertal child can be collected for a urocytogram. A first morning urine specimen is centrifuged and the sediment is spread on a slide. The cytologist records the percentage of superficial, intermediate, and parabasal cells. Two methods for collection and staining are described by Lencioni and Preeyasombat [5, 6].

CERVICAL MUCUS

An examination of the cervical mucus is another method of evaluating a patient's estrogen status. The cervix is gently swabbed with a large cotton-tipped applicator, and a small sample of cervical mucus is obtained with a long forceps or saline-moistened Q-Tip. Scanty,

Table 1-1. Percentage of Parabasal, Intermediate, and Superficial Cells in the Vaginal Smear

State	Parabasal	Intermediate	Superficial
Childhood	60–90	10–20	0–3
Early puberty	30	50	20
Stage V puberty			
Proliferative phase	0	70	30
Secretory phase	0	80–95	5–20
Pregnancy	0	95	5
Anorexia nervosa (depends on clinical status)	75	25	0
Isosexual precocity	20	50	30
Premature thelarche	60	30	5–10
Premature adrenarche	60–90	10–20	0–3

watery mucus is typical of day **8** or **9** of the menstrual cycle; profuse, clear, elastic mucus is typical of days **14** to **16**. Thick, sticky mucus is characteristic of the secretory phase of the cycle (see Chap. 4).

The mucus is spread on a glass slide and allowed to air dry for **10** to **20** minutes. Under the microscope, beautiful ferning patterns will be seen in the late proliferative phase of the cycle (days **14–16**) (Fig. 1-11). Ferning does not occur in the presence of progesterone. If a patient is two weeks late for her period, a smear with good ferning implies a continued proliferative phase and suggests an anovulatory cycle rather than a pregnancy.

WET PREPARATIONS

The so-called wet preps are useful in defining the etiology of a vaginal discharge. In the prepubertal child, the discharge is collected with a saline-moistened Q-Tip or an eyedropper. In adolescents, a Q-Tip is inserted into the vaginal pool with the speculum in place. The Q-Tip is mixed first with one drop of saline on a glass slide and then with one drop of 10% KOH on another slide. A coverslip is then applied, and the slides are examined under the microscope (low and high dry power).

On the saline slide, trichomonads appear as lively, flagellated organisms, slightly larger than a white blood cell. A saline preparation of a *Hemophilus vaginalis* infection typically shows many refractile bacteria within large epithelial cells (so-called clue cells) and some leukocytes. In contrast, physiological leukorrhea is characterized by

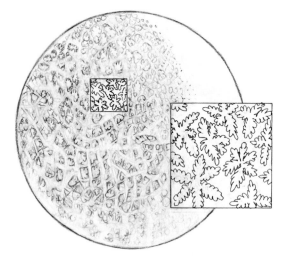

Fig. 1-11. Ferning during late proliferative phase of the normal menstrual cycle.

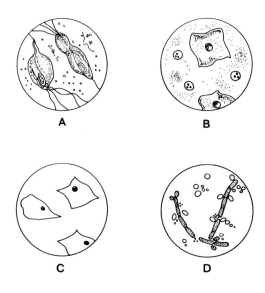

Fig. 1-12. Fresh vaginal smears: (A) Trichomonas, (B) H. vaginalis, (C) *leukorrhea,* (D) Candida (A, B, *and* C *on saline prep;* D *on KOH prep*).

numerous epithelial cells without evidence of inflammation. The KOH preparation allows easy demonstration of the budding hyphae and yeast forms of a monilial vaginitis (Fig. 1-12).

GRAM'S STAIN

In symptomatic gonorrhea, Gram's stain of a vaginal or cervical discharge may reveal polymorphonuclear leukocytes and gram-negative intracellular diplococci; however, because of the presence of saprophytic neisseria in the vagina, only a positive culture is conclusive evidence of this diagnosis.

CULTURES

Sexually active teenage girls should probably have routine cultures for gonorrhea every six months. A Q-Tip is inserted into the cervical os and then streaked directly onto Transgrow, Modified Thayer Martin-Jembec,* or Thayer-Martin media. The use of plain Thayer-Martin plates requires immediate transportation of the culture to a bacteriology laboratory and incubation under increased carbon dioxide tension. Transgrow and Jembec are transport media and can actually be mailed to a laboratory. In high-risk patients, a rectal culture for gonorrhea should also be done, since the recovery rate is thus increased by approximately five percent.

Nickerson's medium (Ortho) is helpful in confirming the presence

* Gibco, Madison, Wis. 53713.

of a monilial vaginitis if the KOH preparation is negative. A sample of the discharge is streaked on the medium, and the tube is incubated in the office at room temperature. The appearance of brown colonies three to seven days later is a positive test for yeast.

PROGESTERONE TEST

The patient is given medroxyprogesterone (Provera), 10 mg orally, for five days, or progesterone-in-oil, 50–100 mg intramuscularly. If the patient has an estrogen-primed endometrium and is not pregnant, she will have a period three to ten days later. Progesterone given orally or intramuscularly is used as a diagnostic test for the evaluation of primary and secondary amenorrhea (see Chap. 6), not as a pregnancy test.

PREGNANCY TESTS

A number of 2-minute urine pregnancy tests are available, including Gravindex*, Pregnosticon Accuspheres,† Pregnosis,‡ and UCG-Slide Test§. The test is done on urine (preferably a first morning urine) and detects human chorionic gonadotropin (HCG) 10–14 days after the first missed period. Simple directions are included in the kits. Tube tests usually done in commercial laboratories or hospitals require 2 hours and become positive about one week earlier than the 2-minute tests. Because quantitation is possible, the tube test may aid in the diagnosis of an ectopic pregnancy (very low levels of HCG) or a molar pregnancy (very high levels of HCG).

False negative urine pregnancy tests occur with early (less than six weeks) and ectopic pregnancies. False positive tests may occur with detergent residues on the glassware and occasionally with heavy proteinuria and certain drugs (e.g., methadone, phenothiazines, or pro-gestational agents) [7].

In many large centers, a new serum pregnancy test, the β-subunit HCG, is available for the detection of early and ectopic pregnancies and the follow-up of patients with molar pregnancies and chorio-carcinoma. Quantitation of extremely low levels of HCG is possible.

BUCCAL SMEAR

The patient is asked to rinse her mouth with water, and a tongue depressor is then scraped along the buccal mucosa. The material is streaked on a glass slide, which is immediately placed in a $3:1$ methanol–acetic acid solution or Pap fixative. The cytologist looks

---

* Ortho Diagnostics, Inc., Route 202, Raritan, N.J. 08869.
† Organon, Inc., 375 Mt. Pleasant Ave., West Orange, N.J. 07052.
‡ Roche Laboratories, Division of Hoffman-La Roche, Inc., Nutley, N.J. 07110.
§ Wampole, P.O. Box 5, Cranbury, N.J. 08512.

for the presence of Barr bodies. In the normal female the chromatin positive material represents the second X chromosome. Since laboratories vary in their "normal counts," a control smear must always be run concurrently. Some laboratories report counts for the normal female in the range of 10–35 percent; others report 19–49 percent. A patient with no Barr bodies is XO or XY; a patient with a low count may be a mosaic (e.g., XX/XO, XX/XY). The presence of two Barr bodies per cell indicates XXX or XXXY. In addition, the size of the chromatin mass can be evaluated by an experienced technician. A small Barr body may signify a deletion of part of the X chromosome; a large Barr body may represent an isochromosome for the long arm of the X chromosome.

Incubating the buccal smear or peripheral blood with quinacrine dye allows demonstration of the Y chromosome by fluorescence (without the necessity of a full karyotype).

Bone Age

The bone age is determined by comparing the x-rays of the patient's wrist and hand (carpal and phalangeal ossification centers) with the standards in Greulich and Pyle [8]. An x-ray of the iliac crest can be used in a similar way. At puberty the epiphysis along the iliac crest undergoes ossification. During adolescence, the ossification progresses lateral to medial, and fusion occurs at 21 to 23 years.

Growth hormone and thyroid deficiencies, glucocorticoid excess, delayed puberty, and malnutrition result in delayed maturation; androgens produce an advanced bone age. The bone age will not advance beyond 13 years in the absence of sex steroids (for example, sexual infantilism associated with Turner's syndrome).

Basal Body Temperature Charts

The basal body temperature chart is used primarily for infertility patients. The patient is instructed to take her temperature every morning as soon as she awakes. For accurate recording, a basal body thermometer is kept at the bedside, and the patient is told "not to go to the bathroom" or "even to wiggle" before the temperature is taken. The temperature is then recorded on a special chart. The typical ovulatory and anovulatory cycles are shown in Figure 1-13.

Although the physician may be curious as to whether the 15- or 16-year-old teenager with oligomenorrhea or Turner's mosaicism XX/XO (and gonadal function) has ovulatory cycles, excessive concern about future fertility may lead to an unwanted pregnancy. In most cases the diagnostic workup is more appropriate at age 18 or 19 or at the time when the patient herself voices concern about her fertility.

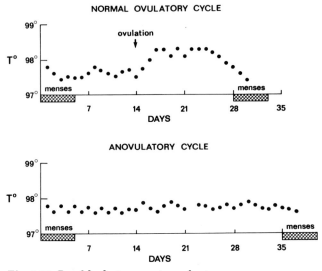

Fig. 1-13. Basal body temperature charts.

REFERENCES

1. Huffman, J.   Gynecologic examination of the premenarcheal child. *Pediatr. Ann.* 3:6, 1974.
2. Capraro, V.   Gynecologic examination in children and adolescents. *Pediatr. Clin. North Am.* 19(3):511, 1972.
3. Capraro, V., and Capraro, E.   Vaginal aspirate studies in children. *Obstet. Gynecol.* 37:462, 1971.
4. Green, T.   *Gynecology: Essentials of Clinical Practice* (3rd ed.). Boston: Little, Brown, 1977.
5. Lencioni, L. J., and Staffieri, J.   Urocytogram diagnosis of sexual precocity. *Acta Cytol.* (Baltimore) 13:302, 1969.
6. Preeyasombat, C., and Kenny, F.   Urocytogram in normal children and various abnormal conditions. *Pediatrics* 38:436, 1966.
7. Urine pregnancy tests.   *Med. Lett. Drugs Ther.* 17:2, 1975.
8. Greulich, W. W., and Pyle, S.   *Radiographic Atlas of Skeletal Development of the Hand and Wrist.* Stanford, Calif.: Stanford University Press, 1959.

SUGGESTED READING

Heald, F. (Ed.).   *Adolescent Gynecology.* Baltimore: Williams & Wilkins, 1966.
Huffman, J.   *The Gynecology of Childhood and Adolescence.* Philadelphia: Saunders, 1969.

2. Ambiguous Genitalia in the Newborn

Although most clinicians do not frequently see an infant with ambiguous genitalia at birth, the need to assess the situation as quickly as possible makes this subject essential. Any deviation from the normal appearance of male or female genitalia should prompt investigation, since apparent male or female external genitals may be associated with the gonads and genotype of the opposite sex, e.g., the male with feminizing testicular syndrome and the markedly virilized female with congenital adrenocortical hyperplasia (CAH). Even slight doubt that arises in the initial newborn examination should be pursued systematically to prevent the possibility of later confusion. Bilateral cryptorchidism, unilateral cryptorchidism with incomplete scrotal fusion or hypospadias, and clitoromegaly require evaluation.

DETERMINING SEX ASSIGNMENT

When the physician finds an infant with ambiguous genitalia, the parents should be reassured that they have a healthy baby but that because the external genital development is incomplete, tests are necessary to determine the sex. A straightforward explanation of the factors necessary for normal sexual development in utero may be helpful. Clearly, most parents will react with dismay and anxiety; they should be reassured that tests will show the cause of the problem and whether their baby is a girl or a boy. The possibility of an intersex disorder (hermaphroditism) should not be raised at this time. Speculation about possible sex assignment should be kept to a minimum; it is not helpful for the physician to say, "I think it's a girl," or "I think it's a boy." The parents should be told that within a few days, or at most one to two weeks, a definite answer will be possible. Some parents will prefer to give their infant a name appropriate for either a girl or a boy (e.g., Frances, Leslie, Bobby); others will prefer to wait and use the names they had previously selected for a boy or girl.

Although a diagnosis of the patient's condition requires knowledge of the genotype (buccal smear with Y fluorescence and karyotype), assignment of sex is based on other criteria as well. The first issue is fertility. The female with CAH may be virilized at birth, yet with normal ovaries and uterus she is potentially capable of bearing children. Thus, management including surgery must aim at a female role. When fertility is not possible, as with mixed gonadal dysgenesis (MGD) or male pseudohermaphroditism, decisions are based on surgical requirements for reconstruction of the external genitals. In general, surgical techniques are more suited to a clitorectomy and later the creation of a vagina than to the construction of a normal male phallus. Once the decision as to sex assignment is made, the physician should help the parents accept their infant as a normal male or a normal female. As long as attitudes toward the child's sex remain unequivocal, the child usually assumes his/her gender role without difficulty regardless of the genotype.

REVIEW OF EMBRYOGENESIS

Prior to the seventh week of gestation, the fetal gonads are sexually bipotential. Differentiation of the gonad to a testis requires a Y chromosome; differentiation to an ovary requires two X chromosomes. Thus, the patient with gonadal dysgenesis (XO) has neither an ovary nor a testis, but rather has *streak gonads*. Male internal and external genital development depends on a functioning testis. Female genital development occurs in the absence of a testis, so a patient with XX (normal female) or XO (Turner's syndrome) has a uterus, fallopian tubes, vagina, and female external genitalia. An outline of normal development is shown in Figures 2-1 and 2-2.

The fetal testis produces two substances: (1) a müllerian-inhibiting substance, which acts locally to prevent the development of the tubes, uterus, and upper vagina, and (2) testosterone, which is responsible for the development of normal male external genitalia and the wolffian system (vas deferens, seminal vesicles, epididymis). By the twelfth week of gestation, the genital tubercle has formed into the penis, and the genital swellings have fused to form the scrotum. Thus, if the testis is present but inadequate through the tenth to twelfth week of gestation, the internal genitalia may be a mixture of müllerian and wolffian structures while the external genitalia are ambiguous (so-called dysgenetic male pseudohermaphroditism). If the testes function until the sixteenth week of gestation and then disappear, the internal and external genitalia will be male except for bilateral cryptorchidism and possible small phallus (so-called congenital anorchia).

The patient with MGD (e.g., XO/XY with a streak gonad on one side and a testis on the other) may have a mixture of müllerian and wolffian structures (e.g., a uterus, tubes, and perhaps a vas deferens). Approximately one-half of patients with MGD have ambiguous genitalia at birth; 26 out of 36 patients in Federman's series [1] were raised as females. Although the intraabdominal testis in MGD does not seem to function adequately to suppress the müllerian structures internally or to virilize the external genitalia completely, it is known

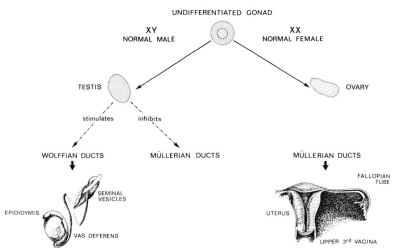

Fig. 2-1. Internal genital differentiation in utero.

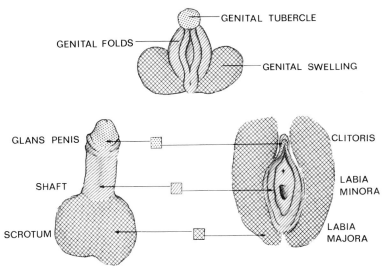

Fig. 2-2. External genital differentiation in utero.

to be capable of producing androgen levels sufficient to cause unwanted virilization of the female at puberty. Perhaps in this situation, testicular differentiation in utero is late and the internal and external structures are no longer sensitive to the local and hormonal effects.

True hermaphroditism does not fit neatly into these hypotheses, for in spite of the fact that 80 percent of such patients have 46/XX leukocyte karyotypes, both ovarian and testicular tissue are present. Internal and external differentiation varies considerably; some patients are almost normal females, others are males with hypospadias, and many have ambiguous genitalia. In the past, most have been raised as males, but at adolescence three-fourths of these patients develop gynecomastia and one-half menstruate.

Patients with testicular feminization (XY), although usually presenting as normal females in the newborn period, are interesting because their testes function normally to inhibit müllerian structures (no tubes, uterus, or upper vagina) and to produce testosterone, but the end-organs are totally unresponsive to androgens. Although testicular feminization represents one end of the spectrum of male pseudo-hermaphroditism, other patients with partial enzymatic blocks of androgen synthesis or variable sensitivity to normal levels of androgen may present with ambiguous genitalia as neonates.

In the absence of testicular function (genotype XX or XO), the müllerian ducts differentiate into the uterus, fallopian tubes, upper one-third of the vagina, and the genital tubercle, folds, and swellings form the normal female external genitalia. However, in the normal XX female, the presence of androgen either from a fetal source (CAH) or a maternal source (certain drugs, maternal CAH, or a virilizing tumor) will alter the external but not the internal genitalia. Progestins such as ethisterone (Pranone*) and norethindrone (Norlutin) and androgens given prior to the fourteenth week of gestation cause labial fusion and clitoromegaly; such therapy after the fourteenth week is only capable of causing clitoromegaly.

Thus, from this brief review of embryogenesis, it is clear that many important disorders are responsible for ambiguous genitalia in the newborn period.

ASSESSMENT OF THE NEONATE

The initial evaluation of the neonate includes a careful history, physical examination, buccal smear with Y fluorescence (and karyotype), and urinary and serum hormone analyses. X-ray contrast studies and surgical evaluation are often necessary to establish the final diagnosis and appropriate sex assignment (Fig. 2-3).

---

* Pranone is no longer commercially available but was widely used in the past.

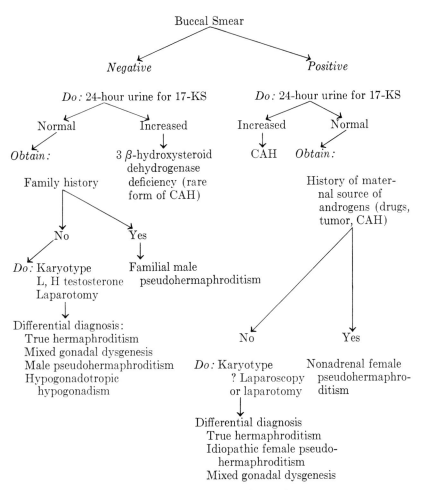

Fig. 2-3. Evaluation of ambiguous genitalia in the newborn.

HISTORY

A careful history should be obtained from the parents regarding:

1. Other family members, especially siblings, with CAH. This diagnosis may be missed in males because the only physical sign is increased scrotal rugation and pigmentation. Thus the history may reveal only a male sibling who died in early infancy with vomiting and dehydration (not recognized as secondary to adrenal insufficiency).
2. Aunts or other relatives with amenorrhea and infertility (suggestive of male pseudohermaphroditism).

3. Maternal ingestion of any drugs during pregnancy, especially Pranone, Norlutin, or androgens.
4. Maternal history of virilization or CAH.

PHYSICAL EXAMINATION

The physical examination of the infant should include measurement of the clitoris/penis and notation of the site of the urethra (perineal vs. penile), fusion of the labioscrotal folds, and the presence of gonads in the scrotum or in the inguinal rings. A rectal exam should be done to assess the presence of a uterus. Because of in utero stimulation by placental estrogen, the uterus is often easily palpable at birth.

LABORATORY TESTS

The important laboratory tests include a buccal smear with Y fluorescence (karyotype later) and a 24-hour urine test for 17-ketosteroids or pregnanetriol. The buccal smear can be done immediately, although low counts are seen in the first two days of life. Few normal females have counts less than 5 percent but many have counts lower than 20 percent; thus a mosaic may be missed. A repeat buccal smear on the third or fourth day of life is indicated if counts are borderline [2]. Staining with a quinacrine dye will pick up the presence of "Y" line.

Collection of the 24-hour urine for 17-ketosteroids can be started immediately. A small metabolic bed is helpful for accurate collections. A 24-hour excretion greater than 3 mg is practically diagnostic of CAH; only very rarely is an adrenal tumor present. An excretion of less than 0.5 mg/24 hours excludes the diagnosis (see Appendix 1). However, normal females occasionally excrete up to 2.0 mg/24 hours for the first one to two weeks of life; after that, greater than 1.0 mg/24 hours) is abnormal. Serum should be sent to an endocrine laboratory for measurement of 17-hydroxyprogesterone (elevated in 21-hydroxylase deficiency). Additional evidence in favor of the diagnosis of CAH is provided by increased urinary pregnanetriol (greater than 0.5 mg/24 hours). In Figure 2-4 the pathways of steroid biosynthesis are reviewed.

THE CHROMATIN-POSITIVE NEWBORN

As is shown in Figure 2-3, the differential diagnosis of chromatin-positive patients includes:

1. Congenital adrenocortical hyperplasia
2. Female pseudohermaphroditism
   a. Due to drugs
   b. Due to maternal CAH or a virilizing tumor
   c. Idiopathic
3. True hermaphroditism
4. Mixed gonadal dysgenesis (XX/XY)

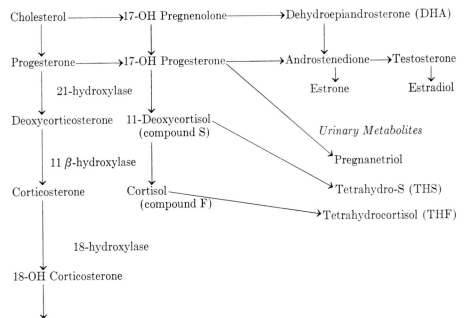

Cholesterol ⟶ 17-OH Pregnenolone ⟶ Dehydroepiandrosterone (DHA)

Progesterone ⟶ 17-OH Progesterone ⟶ Androstenedione ⟶ Testosterone

21-hydroxylase   Estrone   Estradiol

Deoxycorticosterone   11-Deoxycortisol
(compound S)   *Urinary Metabolites*

11 β-hydroxylase   Pregnanetriol

Corticosterone   Cortisol   Tetrahydro-S (THS)
(compound F)   Tetrahydrocortisol (THF)

18-hydroxylase

18-OH Corticosterone

Aldosterone

Fig. 2-4. Major pathways of steroid biosynthesis.

Congenital Adrenocortical Hyperplasia

Congenital adrenocortical hyperplasia represents the most common cause of ambiguous genitalia in the chromatin-positive newborn. Because of the variability in enzymatic block, ambiguity may range from slight clitoromegaly to a "male phallus" with fusion and rugation of the labioscrotal folds. The most common enzymes involved are 21-hydroxylase and 11 β-hydroxylase. Because of inadequate cortisol synthesis, adrenocorticotropic hormone (ACTH) increases with resultant increased adrenal androgen production. Salt-losing is seen in about one-third of patients with the 21-hydroxylase deficiency because of a concomitant block in aldosterone secretion and the increased secretion of compounds that are aldosterone antagonists. Babies with more severe virilization tend to be salt-losers (Fig. 2-5). A deficiency of 11 β-hydroxylase is associated with hypertension and moderately increased urinary excretion of pregnanetriol and the reduced metabolites of 11-deoxycortisol and deoxycorticosterone (Tetrahydro-S and Tetrahydro-DOC). A rare form of CAH, 3 β-hydroxysteroid dehydrogenase deficiency, results in severe adrenal insufficiency and increased ACTH levels; however, virilization is quite mild because the block is in the initial steps of hormone synthesis so that only the weak androgen (dehydroepiandrosterone) can be produced in excess.

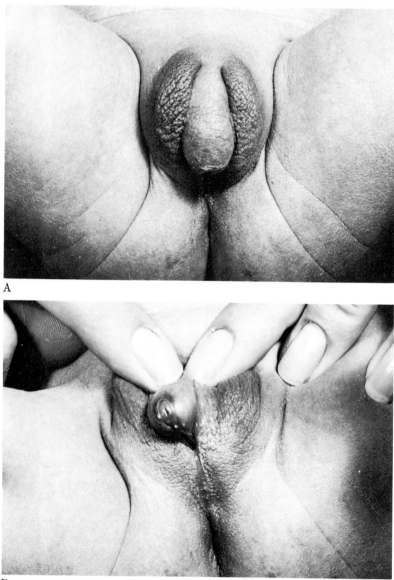

A

B

28

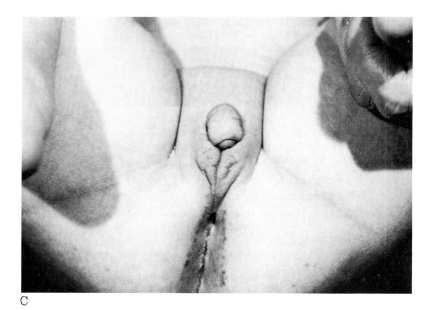

C

Fig. 2-5. Two newborn females presenting with virilization and salt-losing CAH. (A, B) Patient S. C. (C) Patient M. T.

The diagnosis of CAH should be made as soon as possible after birth because of the need for glucocorticoid and salt hormone replacement to prevent dehydration, hyponatremia, and hyperkalemia. Even in highly suspicious cases (sibling with CAH), serum and urine should be collected prior to treatment for the diagnosis. Since salt-losing usually does not occur until the second week of life, studies can be performed without significant risk during the first week, while the baby's weight and electrolytes are monitored in the meantime. If necessary, treatment can then be instituted pending return of the laboratory results. Hydrocortisone, 2.5 mg three times daily (or 13–25 mg/M²/day), is the usual starting dosage. If salt-losing is documented by decreased serum Na$^+$ and increased serum K$^+$ in the second week of life, salt (2–4 gm/day) should be added to the formula and a mineralocorticoid, fludrocortisone acetate (Florinef), 0.05 to 0.1 mg, should be given orally each day. Adjustment of the hydrocortisone dosage is made on the basis of growth parameters (length, weight, skeletal maturation), urinary 17-ketosteroids (maintained at less than 1 mg/24 hours), and if available serum 17-hydroxyprogesterone levels [3]. Overtreatment results in growth retardation, undertreatment in acceleration of the bone age more than the height age and virilization. Illnesses and surgery must be covered by increasing the glucocorticoid dosage.

It should be emphasized that chromatin-positive patients with CAH are females and potentially fertile. Thus, regardless of the appearance of the external genitalia, the sex assignment should be female and surgery later undertaken for (1) extirpation of the clitoris, (2) division of the labioscrotal folds, and (3) creation of an adequate vagina. The first two procedures are usually done after the newborn period, as early in the first year of life as good surgical practice permits. If menstrual drainage is adequate, the third procedure is postponed until the patient is an adolescent and wants to cooperate in the management program. The use of vaginal dilators may be successful in avoiding a surgical vaginoplasty. In cases in which construction is necessary, postoperative use of dilators is usually necessary to keep the vagina patent until the patient has regular sexual relations.

OTHER DIAGNOSES OF CHROMATIN-POSITIVE NEONATES

If an infant is chromatin-positive on buccal smear and has normal 17-ketosteroids, she either has a primary gonadal abnormality or has been exposed to exogenous hormones (androgens or progestins) or a virilizing lesion in the mother. If the drug history is negative, the mother should have a careful physical exam and measurement of urinary 17-ketosteroids and plasma testosterone. In the absence of a history of maternal virilization or hormone ingestion, the infant should have a karyotype and possibly laparoscopy or laparotomy to determine the gonadal causes of the ambiguous genitalia: true hermaphroditism, idiopathic female pseudohermaphroditism, or MGD.

THE CHROMATIN-NEGATIVE NEWBORN

The differential diagnosis of patients with a chromatin-negative buccal smear (and positive Y fluorescence) includes:

1. True hermaphroditism
2. Mixed gonadal dysgenesis
3. Male pseudohermaphroditism
   a. Congenital adrenocortical hyperplasia: $3\,\beta$-hydroxysteroid dehydrogenase, $17\,\alpha$-hydroxylase, and (?) cholesterol $20\,\alpha$-hydroxylase deficiency (all extremely rare)
   b. $5\,\alpha$-Reductase deficiency and other defects in testosterone synthesis (diminished 5-dihydrotestosterone)
   c. Partial androgen insensitivity
   d. Dysgenetic male pseudohermaphroditism (defective testicular gonadogenesis)
4. Hypogonadotropic hypogonadism (Kallman's syndrome)

Severe adrenal insufficiency and incomplete virilization characterize the rare male patient with $3\,\beta$-hydroxysteroid dehydrogenase, $17\,\alpha$-

hydroxylase, and cholesterol 20 α-hydroxylase deficiency. Urinary 17-ketosteroids are elevated with 3 β-hydroxysteroid dehydrogenase deficiency. A history of familial male pseudohermaphroditism (defects in testosterone synthesis or partial androgen insensitivity) in relatives is clearly significant in the differential diagnosis. Palpation of two gonads in the inguinal rings or scrotum favors the diagnosis of male pseudohermaphroditism, although rarely a patient may have a hypothalamic etiology for the micropenis. Cytogenetic studies may be helpful in distinguishing between patients with structural defects or dysgenetic testes (MGD, true hermaphroditism, dysgenetic male pseudohermaphroditism) and those with structurally normal testes (5 α-reductase deficiency, androgen insensitivity). Many patients in the former group have abnormal sex chromosomes with mosaicism; the patients in the latter group have an XY karyotype. Patients with androgen insensitivity have elevated serum testosterone and luteinizing hormone values; patients with diminished 5-dihydrotestosterone have normal testosterone and luteinizing hormone values [4]. Retrograde contrast x-ray studies and laparoscopy or laparotomy are often necessary to establish the final diagnosis. If the patient has a micropenis and testes, sex assignment should be delayed until a one- to three-month course of intramuscular human chorionic gonadotropin (HCG) or local testosterone cream, or both, is tried. If the response is good, a male assignment is made (Fig. 2-6). If the response is poor or if the male phallus is so small that the patient cannot possibly function in the male sexual role, a female identity should be chosen regardless of genotype, for the phallus will not grow at puberty in those with androgen insensitivity.

Decisions for gender identity thus depend on external genitalia and the possibility of future coital adequacy. When the sex assignment is clearly made, the gonads of the opposite sex should be electively removed. For example, the patient with MGD and XO/XY who is given a female sex assignment should have her testis removed to prevent virilization at puberty. Intraabdominal testes in patients with male pseudohermaphroditism and MGD have an increased malignancy risk and thus require prophylactic removal. Hormone therapy is often necessary later for normal pubertal development. In addition, it should be noted that all patients with a genital abnormality should have a careful search for associated anomalies of the urinary tract.

HYPOSPADIAS AND CRYPTORCHIDISM

Hypospadias occurs in newborn males at a ratio of 1 : 600 to 1 : 1800. Although it usually represents an isolated anomaly in an otherwise normal male, it may be the only clue to one of the unusual disorders listed in this chapter. If hypospadias occurs with cryptorchidism

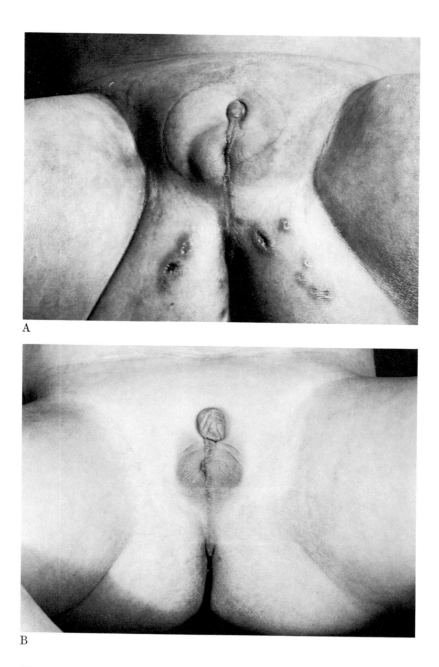

A

B

Fig. 2-6. Infant male with Kallman's syndrome. (A) At age 4 months, M. F. presented with a micropenis and undescended testes. Evaluation revealed a karyotype of XY, and at surgery the testes were brought to the inguinal rings. (B) M. F. at age 1 year. Penile size had increased after a three-month course of intramuscular HCG. M. F. required a repeat orchiopexy at age 12 and HCG therapy to induce pubertal development.

(unilateral or bilateral), any defect in scrotal fusion, or a uterus palpable by rectal exam, a complete evaluation is necessary.

Cryptorchidism should also raise questions. If one testis is absent but the genitalia are otherwise completely normal, a rectal examination should be done to rule out the remote possibility of the existence of a uterus and the diagnosis of an intersex state. If a uterus is not palpated, no further workup is then indicated. If both testes are missing but the genitalia still appear to be those of a normal male, a buccal smear and hormonal analysis should be done to rule out CAH. If the buccal smear is chromatin-negative and the genitals adequate for male function, the infant should be raised as a male; laparotomy to search for the testes can be delayed. Some of these patients have bilateral undescended testes that are capable of function; others have congenital anorchia in which the testes presumably functioned at least until the sixteenth week of gestation and then disappeared. Serum-luteinizing hormone and follicle-stimulating hormone may be elevated early in life in the latter patients, indicating the agonadal state; testosterone therapy at puberty is necessary for the development of secondary sexual characteristics.

REFERENCES

1. Federman, D. *Abnormal Sexual Development*. Philadelphia: Saunders, 1968.
2. Smith, D. W., et al. Lower incidence of sex chromatin in buccal smears of newborn females. *Pediatrics* 30:707, 1962.
3. Hughes, I., and Winter, J. The applications of a serum 17-OH progesterone radioimmunoassay to the diagnosis and management of congenital adrenal hyperplasia. *J. Pediatr.* 88:766, 1976.
4. Donahoe, P., and Hendren, W. Evaluation of the newborn with ambiguous genitalia. *Pediatr. Clin. North Am.* 23(2):361, 1976.

SUGGESTED READING

Capraro, V., Crigler, J., and Huffman, J. Alternative Points of View in the Diagnosis and Management of Ambiguous Sexual Development. In D. Reid and C. Christian (Eds.), *Controversy in Obstetrics and Gynecology*. Philadelphia: Saunders, 1974.
DiGeorge, A. Disorders of the Adrenal Glands. In W. Nelson (Ed.), *Textbook of Pediatrics* (10th ed.). Philadelphia: Saunders, 1975.
Grumbach, M., and Van Wyk, J. Disorders of Sex Differentiation. In R. Williams (Ed.), *Textbook of Endocrinology* (5th ed.). Philadelphia: Saunders, 1974.

3. Vulvovaginal Problems in the Prepubertal Child

VULVOVAGINITIS

Vulvovaginitis is a common complaint in the prepubertal child. The proximity of the vagina to the anus and the thin, atrophic vaginal mucosa make the young child particularly susceptible to vulvovaginal infections with a mixed bacterial flora. After the child reaches the age of 3, mothers tend not to supervise bathing and toilet functions as closely as before, so that perineal hygiene is often inadequate. Young girls may inadvertently wipe feces across the vagina in a back-to-front motion. Moreover, the prepubertal child lacks the protection of the thick labial fat pads and pubic hair of the adolescent and is apt to spend much of her time sitting on the ground and in sandboxes, which are sources of vaginal irritation. Pinworm infestations are common in preschool and school children, and the anal scratching may contaminate the vaginal area with a variety of organisms; rarely an adult pinworm may find its way into the vagina and cause irritation and discharge. Bubble baths and harsh soaps may cause vulvitis and a secondary vaginitis. Tight-fitting, nonabsorbent nylon underpants may result in maceration and infection, especially in hot weather, similar to the diaper dermatitis seen in infants who wear infrequently changed cloth diapers or plastic-covered paper diapers. A vaginal discharge is sometimes seen with systemic infections such as measles, scarlet fever, and chickenpox.

True vulvovaginitis should not be confused with physiological leukorrhea. Newborns and pubescent girls often have copious secretions secondary to the effect of estrogen on the vaginal mucosa. In newborns, since maternal estrogen is responsible for the discharge, the leukorrhea disappears within two to three weeks after birth. The treatment of the pubertal child with leukorrhea is discussed in Chapter 8.

Obtaining the History

In the usual case of vulvovaginitis, the mother brings her daughter to the physician with complaints of discharge, dysuria, or pruritus. A complete history should be obtained prior to the examination. The physician should elicit the quantity, duration, and type of the discharge, perineal hygiene, recent use of medications or bubble baths, symptoms of anal pruritus (associated with pinworm infestation), and recent infections in the patient or family. The discharge may be copious and purulent, or it may be thin and mucoid. The history of a bloody, foul-smelling discharge should alert the physician to the possibility of a foreign body or a necrotic tumor. An odorless bloody discharge may characterize vulvar irritation or trauma, a vaginal or uterine tumor, or precocious puberty. A history of recent infections is important because, for example, a group A β-hemolytic *Streptococcus* vaginitis may follow a streptococcal upper respiratory infection in the child or mother. The child should always be asked to demonstrate how she wipes herself after using the toilet, for her method may not resemble the mother's teaching.

PHYSICAL EXAMINATION

The physical examination of the prepubertal child is described in Chapter 1, p. 2. In most cases of vulvovaginitis, the only findings are a scanty mucoid discharge and an erythematous introitus. The etiology is usually traced to poor perineal hygiene, which results in an infection with a mixed bacterial flora—*Escherichia coli, Staphylococcus, Streptococcus, Proteus,* and *Pseudomonas.* Cultures are unnecessary if the condition responds promptly to the measures listed at the end of this section. Although visualization of the vagina and cervix in the knee-chest position is optimal and usually easily accomplished, this examination is not essential (especially if anesthesia is required) if mild symptoms improve within two to three weeks.

Laboratory tests

If the discharge is persistent or purulent, Gram's stain and culture should be done. As mentioned in Chapter 1, a soft plastic eyedropper (Clinitest* dropper) or a glass eyedropper with plastic tubing attached [1] can be gently inserted through the hymen to aspirate secretions. If only scanty amounts of discharge are obtained, one drop can be placed in Brain Heart Infusion (BHI)† broth. If the discharge is copious, cultures should be planted on blood, McConkey's, and Thayer-Martin (or Transgrow†) media. Wet preparations should be examined for yeast and *Trichomonas,* both rare in the prepubertal child. In fact, the presence of a monilial vulvovaginitis should prompt a urinalysis to exclude diabetes mellitus. The presence of pinworms can be confirmed by asking the mother to touch the perianal area with Scotch tape or a "pinworm paddle" as soon as the child awakes in the morning. The tape is affixed to a slide and then examined under the microscope for the characteristic eggs (Fig. 3-1).

TREATMENT

In spite of this further evaluation, nonspecific vaginitis remains the diagnosis in most cases. Specific vaginitis probably accounts for less than 20 percent of cases in young children. Primary treatment should

---

* Ames Co., Division of Miles Laboratories, Elkart, Ind. 46514.
† Scott Laboratories, Fiskeville, R.I. 02823.

37

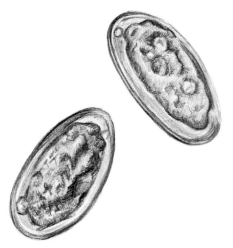

Fig. 3-1. Pinworm eggs (Enterobius vermicularis).

aim at improved perineal hygiene. Systemic antibiotics should be instituted when a specific pathogen is demonstrated, e.g., gonococcus,
group A β-hemolytic *Streptococcus*, pneumococcus. Usually, however,
a mixed culture of bowel flora is reported. If the vaginitis in these
cases is not brought under control with local hygiene in three or four
weeks, two treatment regimens may be tried (either together or in
sequence): (1) a course of oral antibiotics for 10–14 days, or (2) an
estrogen-containing cream applied locally for two to three weeks.
Antibiotics are sometimes effective, at least temporarily, in persistent
cases. Estrogen creams usually give considerable improvement because
the vaginal mucosa becomes thickened and acidic and is thus more
resistant to bacterial invasion. The mother and child should be
warned of the side effects of prolonged local estrogen treatment—breast
soreness and vulvar pigmentation. Fortunately, both are reversible
after the cream is discontinued.

In patients with a persistent vaginal discharge, vaginal examination
in the knee-chest position or by vaginoscopy is clearly necessary to
rule out a tumor or foreign body. Recurrent vaginal discharge often occurs in patients with reflux of urine (especially if infected) into the
vagina. The rare situation of an ectopic ureter or rectovaginal fistula
should also at least be considered.

SUMMARY OF THERAPY

Nonspecific vulvovaginitis (80 percent of cases)

GENERAL MEASURES

1. Good perineal hygiene (including wiping from front to back after
   bowel movements).

2. Frequent changes of white cotton underpants to absorb discharge.
3. Avoidance of bubble baths and harsh soaps.
4. Sitz baths two or three times daily with plain warm water. The vulva should be gently washed with a mild, nonscented soap (Basis, Oilatum, Castile). The bath should be followed by careful drying (patting, not rubbing). Optimally the child should then lie with her legs spread apart for approximately ten minutes to complete the drying. A nonscented talcum powder (e.g., baby powder) can be applied to the vulva.

FOR ACUTE SEVERE EDEMATOUS VULVITIS

1. Sitz baths every 4 hours (with plain water or with a small amount of baking soda added). Soap should not be used, and the vulva should be air dried.
2. Witch hazel pads (Tucks) give soothing relief and may be used in place of toilet paper for wiping. After the acute phase of one to two days, the sitz baths can be alternated every 4 hours with painting on a bland solution such as calamine or a mixture of zinc oxide (15%), talc (15%), and glycerine (10%) in water [2].
3. In the subacute phase, if pruritus is a problem, one of the following creams can be applied locally: (1) hydrocortisone cream 1% with or without the addition of nystatin (Mycostatin) cream, (2) neomycin sulfate with hydrocortisone 1% (Neo-Cortef cream 1%), (3) iodochlorhydroxyquin with hydrocortisone (Vioform-Hydrocortisone cream), or (4) Mycolog cream.
   (*Note:* Vioform can cause a false positive ferric chloride test for phenylketonuria. Vioform, Neo-Cortef, and Mycolog should not be used under occlusive dressings for prolonged periods because of possible sensitization.

   Occasionally an oral medication to lessen pruritus is indicated, i.e., hydroxyzine hydrochloride (Atarax), 2 mg/kg/day in four doses, or diphenhydramine HCl (Benadryl), 5 mg/kg/day in four doses.

FOR PERSISTENT NONSPECIFIC VULVOVAGINITIS

1. Broad spectrum antibiotics, such as ampicillin, 50 mg/kg/day in four doses, *or*
2. Tetracycline, 25 mg/kg/day (if over age 8) in four doses, *and/or*
3. Estrogen-containing creams (Premarin cream), applied nightly to the vulva or with a Q-Tip dabbed into the vagina for two or three weeks, and then every other night for two weeks. A repeat course may be necessary.

Specific vaginitis (20 percent of cases)

GENERAL MEASURES

Good perineal hygiene and sitz baths as described above.

FOR GONOCOCCUS

See p. 115.

FOR GROUP A β-HEMOLYTIC STREPTOCOCCUS OR PNEUMOCOCCUS

1. Penicillin, 125–250 mg orally four times daily for 10 days.
2. Alternatively, erythromycin, 30–50 mg/kg/day orally in three or four doses (up to 250 mg three times daily).

FOR TRICHOMONAS

Metronidazole (Flagyl), 125 mg orally three times daily for five days or 1–2 gm orally (all in one dose).

FOR PINWORMS (ENTEROBIUS VERMICULARIS)

1. Mebendazole (Vermox), one chewable 100-mg tablet (regardless of weight), *or*
2. Pyrantel pamoate (Antiminth) oral suspension, 50 mg/ml, given 11 mg/kg, or more simply 1 ml/10 pounds (maximum 20 ml), as a single dose orally, *or*
3. Pyrvinium pamoate (Povan), 5 mg/kg orally as a single dose (may cause red staining).

FOR CANDIDA

1. Nystatin ointment or cream (Mycostatin) applied to the vulva three times daily for two weeks. (An ointment is preferred for dry, scaly lesions; a cream for moist lesions.)
2. Sitz baths (with a pinch of baking soda) three times daily.

In persistent cases of *Candida:*

1. Nystatin, 100,000 units orally four times daily.
2. Nystatin (100,000 units/ml), 1 ml instilled into the vagina with a plastic eyedropper three times daily.
3. Check urine for sugar (to rule out diabetes mellitus).

VAGINAL BLEEDING

Vaginal bleeding in the prepubertal child should always be carefully assessed. In the neonate, slight vaginal bleeding is sometimes seen in the first week of life secondary to withdrawal from maternal estrogen. After that, the causes to be considered include vaginitis, trauma, a foreign body, a tumor, precocious puberty, and blood dyscrasias (although rare). A good history and physical examination are important in making the differential diagnosis. Foul-smelling vaginal bleeding may originate from a foreign body or necrotic tumor; odorless vaginal bleeding may signify a tumor, trauma, or precocious puberty. A history of exposure to diethylstilbestrol in utero should prompt vaginoscopy (under anesthesia if necessary) to rule out the rare carcinoma. Acceleration of height and weight or signs of pubertal development before the age of 8 suggest precocious puberty (see Chap. 5). A history of previous foreign bodies in the ears or vagina may implicate another foreign body. Patients with blood dyscrasias typically have other signs of bleeding, such as epistaxis, petechiae, or hematomas.

The physical exam should include a general assessment and a careful gynecological exam. Trauma and vulvovaginitis are usually evident on inspection. It should be remembered that unexplained trauma may be a sign of unsuspected sexual molestation. If excoriations are noted around the anus and vulva, a Scotch tape test should be done to search for pinworms. Visualization of the vagina in the knee-chest position or by vaginoscopy is essential and may reveal small wads of toilet paper, pins, or paper; only rarely will a tumor be found.

Bleeding secondary to vulvitis and trauma should respond promptly to local measures. Removal of foreign bodies is often difficult and usually requires either sedation with Demerol compound* or general anesthesia. In the cooperative patient, soft foreign bodies can often be easily removed by twirling a dry cotton-tipped applicator within the vagina or by gentle irrigation with saline or water using a small urethral catheter attached to an eyedropper. Metallic items such as safety pins can be removed with bayonet forceps. If the child continues to insert small wads of toilet paper into her vagina, substitution of thick witch hazel pads (Tucks) for wiping should be considered. Therapy for tumors depends on the extent of the lesion; referral to a large center is essential.

CONDYLOMA ACUMINATUM

The warty lesions known as condyloma acuminatum are occasionally seen in the prepubertal child, especially in association with *Trichomonas* vaginitis. Lesions should be biopsied to establish a definitive diagnosis and then treated with cryocautery, electrodessication, or podophyllin (p. 109).

LABIAL ADHESIONS

Labial adhesions usually occur in young girls 2 to 6 years of age. The cause is unknown but may be related to an irritation that erodes the vulvar epithelium, causing the labia to stick together. Occasionally the vaginal orifice is completely covered, causing poor drainage of vaginal secretions. Mothers often become alarmed because the vagina appears "absent."

In mild cases no treatment is necessary because the labia will separate completely with estrogenization at puberty. In cases in which vaginal or urinary drainage is impaired, an estrogen-containing cream

---

* Demerol compound: 25 mg of meperidine, 6.25 mg of chlorpromazine, and 6.25 mg of promethazine per milliliter with a dosage of 0.1 ml/kg (maximum 2 ml), given intramuscularly.

(Premarin cream) should be applied nightly for two weeks. Occasionally a repeat course of therapy is necessary. Forceful separation is generally contraindicated because it is traumatic for the child and may cause the adhesions to form again.

REFERENCES

1. Capraro, V., and Capraro, E.   Vaginal aspirate studies in children. *Obstet. Gynecol.* 37:462, 1971.
2. Altchek, A.   Pediatric vulvovaginitis. *Pediatr. Clin. North Am.* 19(3):559, 1972.

SUGGESTED READING

Altchek, A.   Vulvovaginal irritation and discharge in children. *Surg. Clin. North Am.* 40:1071, 1960.
Huffman, J.   *The Gynecology of Childhood and Adolescence.* Philadelphia: Saunders, 1969.

4. The Physiology of Puberty

A good understanding of the physiology of puberty and menarche is essential as a background to the diagnosis of precocious puberty in the child and the common menstrual and growth problems of the adolescent. This chapter presents a brief discussion of these issues; more detailed information can be found in the references at the end of the chapter.

HORMONAL CHANGES IN PUBERTY

During childhood, the sex hormones have a negative feedback to the hypothalamus; small amounts of estrogen suppress gonadotropins. In addition, the gonad in the prepubertal girl is suppressed; experimentally, the ovary responds poorly to exogenous luteinizing hormone (LH) and follicle-stimulating hormone (FSH). Before the onset of pubertal changes, the hypothalamus produces releasing factors that stimulate the pituitary to release FSH and small amounts of LH, initially as nighttime surges. With time, the ovaries become responsive to the pituitary hormones and begin to produce estrogens. Estrogen is then responsible for the appearance of breast development and for the maturation of the uterus, vagina, and external genitalia. An increase in adrenal androgens is associated with the appearance of pubic and axillary hair (Fig. 4-1). The growth spurt accompanies these changes in steroid hormone production.

STAGES OF BREAST AND PUBIC HAIR DEVELOPMENT

In 1969, Marshall and Tanner recorded the rates of progression of pubertal development of 192 English schoolgirls [1]. These stages can be important guidelines in assessing whether an adolescent is developing normally. The Tanner stages for breast development are (Fig. 4-2):

Stage B1: Preadolescent; elevation of the nipple only.
Stage B2: Breast bud stage; elevation of the breast and nipple as a small mound, enlargement of the areolar diameter.
Stage B3: Further enlargement of the breast and areola with no separation of the contours.
Stage B4: Further enlargement with projection of the areola and nipple to form a secondary mound above the level of the breast.
Stage B5: Mature stage; projection of the nipple only, resulting from recession of the areola to the general contour of the breast.

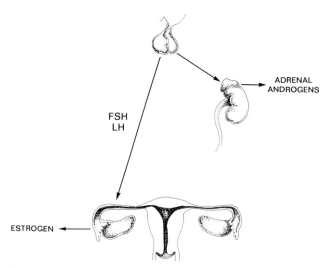

Fig. 4-1. Hormones responsible for the onset of puberty.

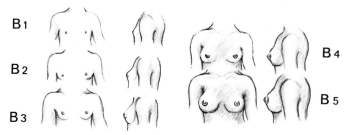

Fig. 4-2. The Tanner stages of human breast maturation. (Adapted from Williams [2].)

45

PH 1   PH 2   PH 3

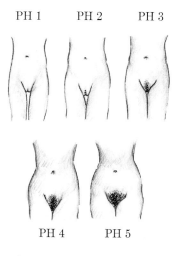

PH 4   PH 5

Fig. 4-3. The Tanner stages for the development of female pubic hair. (Adapted from Williams [2].)

The pubic hair stages are (Fig. 4-3) :

Stage PH1: None.
Stage PH2: Sparse growth of long, straight, only slightly curled hair along the labia.
Stage PH3: Thicker, coarser, and more curled hair extending sparsely over the junction of the pubis.
Stage PH4: Hair is adult in type and spreads over the mons pubis but not to the medial surface of the thighs.
Stage PH5: Hair is spread to the medial surface of the thighs.

The mean age of each stage of puberty is shown in Figure 4-4. Breast development before age 8 would suggest precocious puberty; no breast development by age 14 would suggest delayed development (see Chap. 6).

The appearance of breast development usually corresponds to the onset of the growth spurt and precedes pubic hair growth. However, once pubic hair begins to develop, maturation (stages PH2 to PH5) progresses more rapidly than breast development. In Tanner's series, the mean interval from stages B2 to B5 was 4.2 years and from stages PH2 to PH5, 2.7 years. Thus, it would be extremely unusual for a patient to attain stage 5 breast development without pubic hair development; this would certainly raise the question of testicular feminization syndrome (see Chap. 6). The development of mature pubic hair without any evidence of breast development would suggest

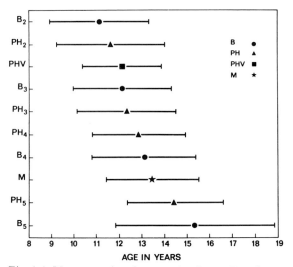

Fig. 4-4. Mean age of each stage of puberty. B = *breast;* PH = *pubic hair;* M = *menarche;* PHV = *peak height velocity. The center of each symbol represents the mean; the length of the symbol is equivalent to two standard deviations on either side of the mean. (Adapted from Marshall and Tanner [1].)*

the presence of androgen alone and would raise the possibility of either an estrogen deficiency or a virilized state.

GROWTH PATTERNS

The growth spurt is dependent on the onset of puberty. Growth charts, such as those illustrated in Figure 4-5, are helpful in evaluating normal development. The inserts on both charts represent velocities, i.e., the peak is at the maximum rate of linear growth and weight gain. The peak height velocity is attained in the majority of teenagers before the Tanner stages B3 and PH2. Figure 4-6 shows the growth chart of a patient with precocious puberty; the early acceleration in height and weight gain at age 2–3 is followed by premature fusion of the epiphyses and attainment of adult height by the age of 10. Figure 4-7 is the growth chart of a patient with delayed development and regional enteritis; normal linear growth is impaired and the patient is relatively underweight for height. Since the timing of the growth spurt during normal development appears to be related to weight and body composition, Frisch [4] has developed a method of predicting the age of the initiation of the growth spurt based on height and weight at age 8.

Skeletal proportions are determined by the rate of pubertal development. The upper/lower (U/L) ratio is approximately 1.0 by age 10.

(L is the distance from the patient's symphysis pubis to the floor, with the patient standing; U is the height minus L.) At puberty, the extremities rapidly increase in length while the vertebral column lengthens more gradually. Initially the U/L ratio may dip to 0.9. As the epiphyses of the legs close, the vertebrae continue to add height and thus the final adult U/L ratio approximates 1.0. In patients with gonadal failure, the lower segment becomes relatively longer because of delayed fusion; thus the U/L ratio may be approximately 0.8. Span (the distance between the fingertips of outstretched arms) usually reflects the same clinical situation; if the span is more than 2 inches greater than the height, the patient has eunuchoid proportions.

MENARCHE

The mean age at menarche in Tanner's series in England was 13.46 ± .46 years, with a range of 9 to 16 years. Zacharias and Wurtman obtained a mean age of menarche among student nurses in the United States of 12.65 ± 1.2 years [5]. Table 4-1 shows that most patients had attained stage 4 breast and pubic hair development at the time of menarche.

In Tanner's series, the mean interval from breast development to menarche was 2.3 ± 0.1 years, but the range was 0.5–5.75 years. A late onset of pubertal development did not appear to change the intervals in the stages of development. Frisch has shown that early and late menarcheal girls have the same *mean* weight of about 47 kg (103½ pounds). She has also established a nomogram for predicting the age of menarche based on height and weight at ages 9 to 13 [4].

In a retrospective series, Zacharias and Wurtman [5, 6] found that the interval between menarche and regular periods was approximately fourteen months and the interval between menarche and painful (presumably ovulatory) periods was approximately twenty-four months. Recent data, however, indicate that ovulatory cycles may begin less than twelve months after the menarche [7].

Table 4-1. Percentage of Patients in Stages 1–5 at Time of Menarche

Stage	Breast (% of patients)	Pubic Hair (% of patients)
1	0	1
2	1	4
3	26	19
4	62	63
5	11	14

Source: Adapted from W. A. Marshall and J. M. Tanner [1].

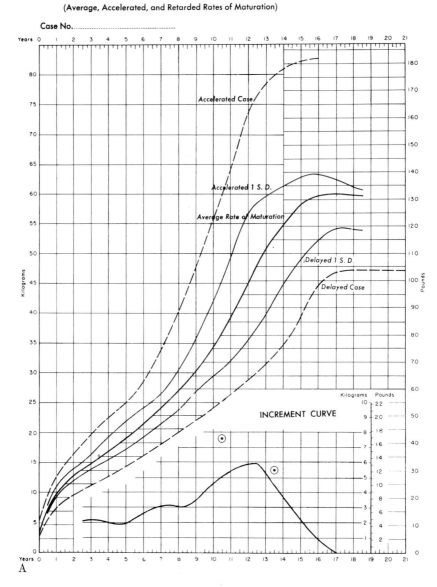

GROWTH CURVES OF WEIGHT BY AGE FOR GIRLS
(Average, Accelerated, and Retarded Rates of Maturation)

Fig. 4-5. Growth charts. (A) Weight, (B) height. (Reproduced from N. Bayley [3], J. Pediatr. 48:187, 1956. By permission of the author and the C. V. Mosby Co.)

GROWTH CURVES OF HEIGHT BY AGE FOR GIRLS
(Average, Accelerated, and Retarded Rates of Maturation)

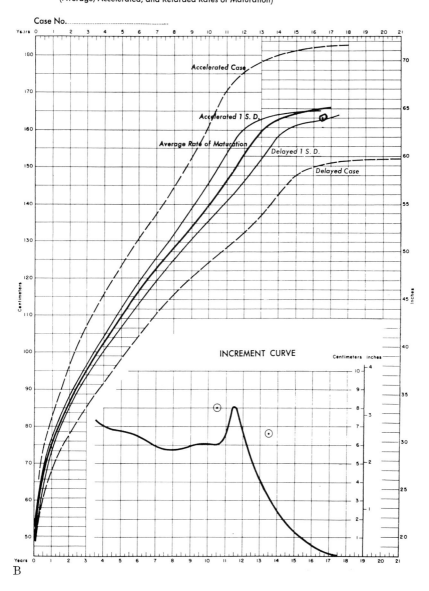

Case No.

Accelerated Case

Accelerated 1 S. D.

Average Rate of Maturation

Delayed 1 S. D.

Delayed Case

INCREMENT CURVE

Centimeters   Inches

Centimeters

Inches

Years

B

49

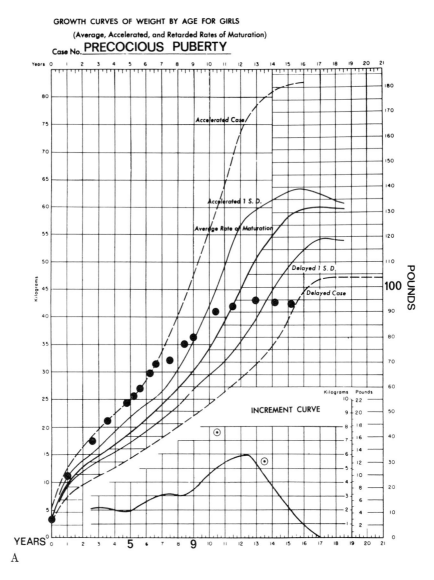

GROWTH CURVES OF WEIGHT BY AGE FOR GIRLS
(Average, Accelerated, and Retarded Rates of Maturation)
Case No. **PRECOCIOUS PUBERTY**

A

Fig. 4-6. Growth charts of patient with idiopathic precocious puberty. (A) Weight, (B) height. (Reproduced from N. Bayley [3], J. Pediatr. 48:187, 1956. By permission of the author and the C. V. Mosby Co.)

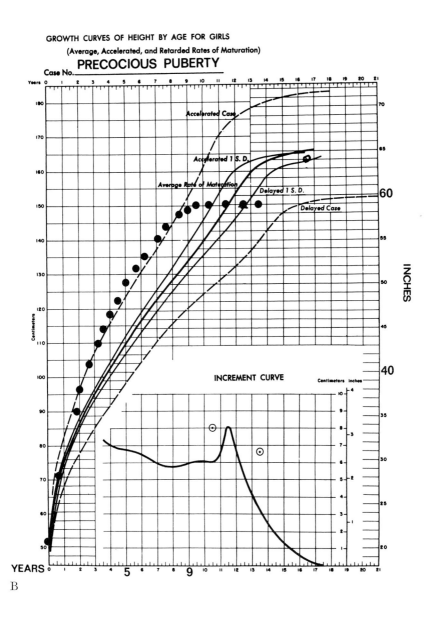

GROWTH CURVES OF HEIGHT BY AGE FOR GIRLS

(Average, Accelerated, and Retarded Rates of Maturation)

PRECOCIOUS PUBERTY

Case No._____

INCHES

INCREMENT CURVE

YEARS

B

51

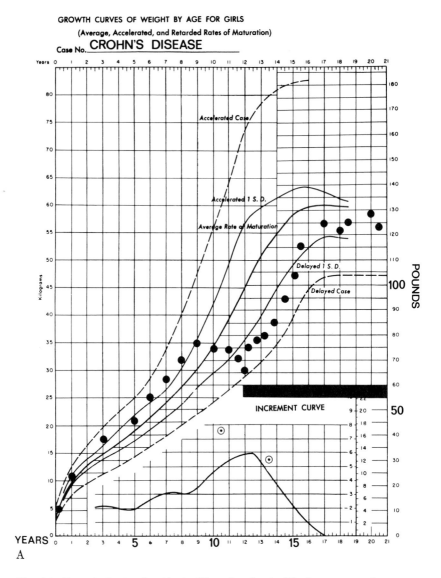

Fig. 4-7. *Growth charts of patient with regional enteritis; bar represents treatment with prednisone. (A) Weight, (B) height. (Reproduced from N. Bayley [3], J. Pediatr. 48:187, 1956. By permission of the author and the C. V. Mosby Co.)*

53

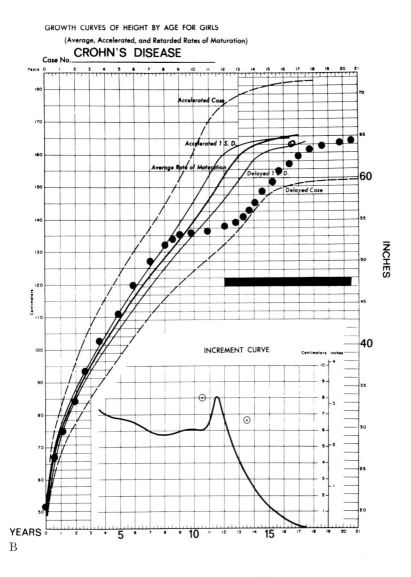

GROWTH CURVES OF HEIGHT BY AGE FOR GIRLS

(Average, Accelerated, and Retarded Rates of Maturation)

CROHN'S DISEASE

Case No._____

B

HORMONE LEVELS IN NORMAL OVULATORY CYCLES

The establishment of ovulatory cycles depends on the maturation of
a positive feedback mechanism in which the rising estrogen levels
trigger an LH surge at midcycle. This means that gonadotropins (FSH
and LH) are released cyclically and tonically in contrast to the tonic
secretion that characterizes the anovulatory cycles of early adolescence
(Fig. 4-8).

The theoretical 28-day cycle can be seen in Figure 4-9. Early in the
cycle, low levels of FSH and LH stimulate the growth of follicles in
the ovaries to produce estrogen. The level of estrogen gradually in-

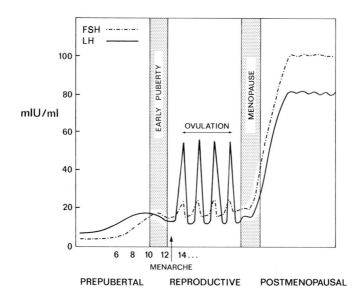

Fig. 4-8. Gonadotropin levels from age 6 to menopause.

creases, resulting in a decreasing FSH (negative feedback) and a slowly increasing LH (predominantly positive feedback). The rising estrogen level produces a proliferative endometrium with thickening of the mucosa and increasing length of the glands. The rapid growth of the "chosen" graafian follicle then leads to a rapid increase in estrogen, which triggers a surge of LH. This surge results in follicular rupture within 16 to 24 hours and expulsion of the oocyte. As is evident in Figure 4-9, there is also a small rise in FSH at midcycle. The mechanism for the rapid decline in LH is unknown, but it may be related to decreasing estrogen levels, depletion of LH stores, or perhaps rising progesterone levels.

Development of the corpus luteum is influenced by LH and follicular rupture. The luteal phase is marked by rising progesterone and estrogen levels, which produce the secretory endometrium character- ized by coiling of the endometrial glands, increased vascularity of the stroma, and increased glycogen content of the epithelial cells. Matura- tion of the endometrium is reached within eight to nine days after ovulation, and then regression begins if fertilization of the ovum does not occur. Without pregnancy and the concomitant rising placen- tal human chorionic gonadotropin, the progesterone and estrogen levels begin to decline. Subsequently, FSH and LH levels begin to rise to start a new cycle. With the waning of progesterone and estrogen the endometrium undergoes necrotic changes in the mucosa, with resulting menstrual bleeding.

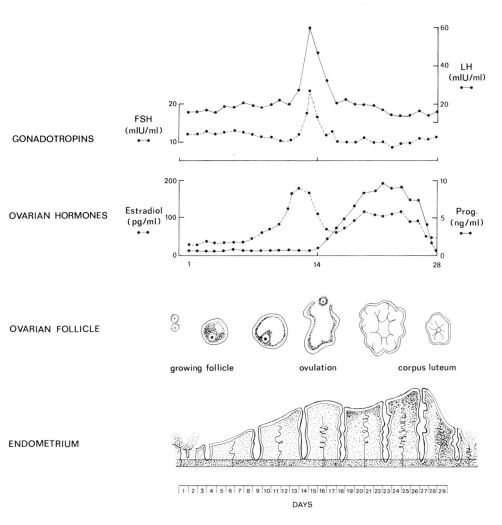

Fig. 4-9. Physiology of the normal ovulatory menstrual cycle: gonadotropins, ovarian hormones, follicular maturation, and endometrial changes.

CLINICAL APPLICATIONS

Understanding the normal cycle is useful in clinical management. In patients with anovulatory cycles, the endometrium remains in the proliferative stage; menstrual periods may be heavy and irregular. Dramatic relief can often be obtained with medroxyprogesterone (Provera) given five days per month to produce a secretory endometrium; three to seven days after the Provera, the patient then has a normal period. In the evaluation of the patient with amenorrhea, a withdrawal flow after intramuscular progesterone implies that the endometrium has been adequately primed with estrogen (see Chap. 6).

Measurement of serum FSH and LH levels by radioimmunoassay is practical and useful. Serum can be sent by the primary care physician to the endocrine laboratory of a teaching hospital or to a reliable commercial laboratory. It is important to remember that laboratories do vary in normal values as well as units per milliliter (mIU/ml or ng/ml). Because gonadotropins are released in pulses, a single random serum value of LH/FSH may not be helpful in distinguishing between low and normal levels of these hormones. In Figure 4-9, the variability of values in normal cycles is evident. Levels of 10 to 25 mIU/ml are in the normal range; consistently low values of 2 to 4 mIU/ml may imply hypothalamic or pituitary hypofunction. An FSH level greater than 50–60 mIU/ml and an LH level greater than 40 mIU/ml in a prepubertal or poorly estrogenized female imply ovarian failure; such high levels are also found in the postmenopausal woman. Gonadotropin-releasing hormone (LHRH) has been recently synthesized and is available in some research centers to study pituitary function. Readers interested in this test are referred to the references listed at the end of this chapter [2, 7] and selected reading on the subject at the end of Chapter 6.

Although measurements of serum estrogen, progesterone, and androgens are possible in specialized laboratories, evaluation of the response of the target organ to these hormones is more practical for the majority of physicians. Pubertal breast development, a pink, succulent vaginal mucosa, and watery cervical mucus imply functioning ovaries and the presence of estrogen. Axillary and pubic hair imply functioning adrenal glands and the presence of androgens. Hirsutism and clitoromegaly are signs of androgen excess and can be evaluated by a few simple laboratory tests.

The assessment of many gynecological problems depends on a careful physical examination (see Chap. 1) combined with a thorough understanding of normal pubertal development. Primary and secondary amenorrhea, menorrhagia, and virilization can then be evaluated in terms of the hypothalamic-ovarian-adrenal axis.

REFERENCES

1. Marshall, W. A., and Tanner, J. M. Variations in pattern of pubertal changes in girls. *Arch. Dis. Child.* 44:291, 1969.
2. Ross, G., and Vande Wiele, R. The Ovaries. In R. Williams (Ed.), *Textbook of Endocrinology* (5th ed.). Philadelphia: Saunders, 1974.
3. Bayley, N. Growth curves of height and weight by age for boys and girls, scaled according to physical maturity. *J. Pediatr.* 48:187, 1956.
4. Frisch, R. E. A method of prediction of age and menarche from height and weight at ages nine through thirteen years. *Pediatrics* 53:384, 1974.
5. Zacharias, L., and Wurtman, R. Age at menarche: Genetic and environmental influences. *N. Engl. J. Med.* 280:868, 1969.
6. Zacharias, L., et al. Sexual maturation in contemporary American girls. *Am. J. Obstet. Gynecol.* 108:833, 1970.

7. Grumbach, M. M., Grave, G. G., and Mayer, F. E. *The Control of the Onset of Puberty*. New York: Wiley, 1974.

SUGGESTED READING

Bayer, L., and Bayley, N. *Growth Diagnosis* (2nd ed.). Chicago: University of Chicago Press, 1976.

Jenner, M. R., et al. Hormonal changes at puberty. *J. Clin. Endocrinol. Metab.* 34:521, 1972.

Kulin, H., and Reiter, E. Gonadotropins during childhood and adolescence: A review. *Pediatrics* 51:260, 1973.

Root, A. Endocrinology of puberty. *J. Pediatr.* 83:1, 187, 1973.

Villee, D. *Human Endocrinology*. Philadelphia: Saunders, 1975.

5. Precocious Puberty

A thorough understanding of the normal progression of puberty (see Chap. 4) is essential in the evaluation of precocious puberty, premature thelarche, and premature adrenarche. It should be recalled that in normal adolescence estrogen is responsible for breast development, for maturation of the external genitalia, vagina, and uterus, and for the menses. An increase in adrenal androgens is associated with the appearance of pubic and axillary hair. Excess androgens of either ovarian or adrenal origin may cause acne, hirsutism, voice changes, increased muscle mass, and clitoromegaly. Thus, precocious puberty in females can be divided into two categories: (1) isosexual precocity, in which the patient has normal pubertal development including menses, and (2) heterosexual precocity, in which the patient has evidence of virilization with or without changes characteristic of a normal puberty.

Premature thelarche is defined as the isolated appearance of breast development; premature adrenarche is the isolated appearance of pubic (and/or axillary) hair without signs of estrogenization. Since, in normal puberty, there may be a dissociation between the time of appearance of sexual hair and breast development, premature thelarche or adrenarche may be the first sign of a true precocious puberty. Because most cases of precocity require fairly sophisticated endocrine studies, referral to an endocrinologist is often necessary.

ISOSEXUAL PRECOCIOUS PUBERTY

Over the past century, the age of onset of pubertal development and menarche has steadily declined in the United States, perhaps in part because of improved nutrition. Currently sexual development (culminating in menarche) before age 8 is defined as "precocious." Isosexual precocious puberty can be divided into two categories on the basis of etiology: true isosexual precocity and isosexual pseudoprecocity.

In true isosexual precocity the stimulus for development arises in the hypothalamus and pituitary gland. In response to rising luteinizing hormone (LH) and follicle-stimulating hormone (FSH) levels, the ovaries produce estrogen. The young girl develops breasts and pubic and axillary hair and begins menstruation, sometimes not in the usual sequence. With the establishment of the cyclic midcycle LH peak, the child becomes potentially fertile.

In isosexual pseudoprecocity an ovarian tumor or cyst produces estrogen autonomously. The fluctuating estrogen levels result in sexual development and anovulatory menses.

In over 80 percent of cases of isosexual precocious puberty, the hypothalamic-pituitary axis is activated prematurely for unknown reasons. Interestingly, approximately 80 percent of patients with idiopathic precocious puberty have abnormal electroencephalograms (EEGs), suggesting a neuroendocrine dysfunction [1]. In addition, the occasional finding of a small hamartoma adjacent to the hypothalamus at incidental post mortem suggests that at least some of the idiopathic cases have a defined central nervous system (CNS) cause.

Despite the high frequency of constitutional or idiopathic precocious puberty, this diagnosis cannot be made without a thorough evaluation and exclusion of the organic disorders [2, 3, 4, 5] listed below:

1. Cerebral disorders (5–10 percent of cases): brain tumor (glioma, pinealoma, hamartoma); postinfectious encephalitis; hydrocephalus; McCune-Albright syndrome (polyostotic fibrous dysplasia, facial asymmetry, and café-au-lait spots with irregular borders); tuberous sclerosis; neurofibromatosis.
2. Ovarian tumors (5 percent of cases): Approximately 60 percent of ovarian tumors that cause sexual precocity are granulosa cell tumors; the remainder are arrhenoblastomas, lipoid cell tumors, thecomas, and cysts.
3. Gonadotropin-producing tumors (rare): Choriocarcinoma is usually rapidly fatal, and thus most patients have only early signs of breast development and pubic hair at the time of diagnosis.
4. Hypothyroidism (rare).
5. Iatrogenic disorders (rare): e.g., the use of estrogen-containing creams and medications.

PATIENT EVALUATION

The initial evaluation of the patient with precocious development should include a careful history and physical examination. Of particular importance is a history of birth trauma, encephalitis, personality changes, seizures, headaches, visual symptoms, abdominal pain, urinary and bowel symptoms, or use of medications and creams. The age of menarche of sisters, mother, and grandmothers should be recorded, and a family history of neurofibromatosis, tuberous sclerosis, or McCune-Albright syndrome should be noted. Vaginal bleeding may be the first sign of precocity in the McCune-Albright syndrome, but it has been noted in idiopathic cases as well. Irregular bleeding occurs in patients with both true precocity and pseudoprecocity. Growth charts should be brought up to date, since the growth spurt often correlates with the onset of development in precocious puberty. The photograph and growth charts of a typical patient with idiopathic precocious puberty are shown in Figure 5-1.

The physical examination should include a careful neurological assessment, visualization of the optic discs for evidence of papilledema, evaluation of visual fields by confrontation, and measurement of the head circumference. It is extremely important to note the degree of breast development and pubic and axillary hair and the appearance of the vaginal mucosa. Signs of virilization, clitoromegaly, or voice changes should alert the examiner to the possibility of heterosexual precocity (see p. 65). If the child is approached in a relaxed manner, a good rectal exam is often possible. Ovarian masses, when present, are usually easily palpable. If an adequate examination is not feasible, a rectal and vaginal examination under anesthesia should be scheduled.

The necessary laboratory tests include:

1. Skull x-ray films
2. Hand and wrist x-ray films for bone age
3. Vaginal smear or urocytogram for estrogen
4. EEG
5. Urine pregnancy test for human chorionic gonadotropin (HCG)
6. Serum FSH and LH levels, and if available estrone, estradiol, progesterone, testosterone, and 17-hydroxyprogesterone levels
7. Twenty-four-hour urine specimen for 17-ketosteroids and pregnanediol

The bone age will always become significantly greater than the height age in patients with precocious puberty. Although a girl may appear tall at the initial evaluation, she may eventually end up quite short for her age because of premature epiphyseal closure. Approximately 50 percent of patients have a final height less than 5 feet. The younger the patient is at the onset of puberty, the shorter she is likely to be. A retarded bone age suggests the rare diagnosis of hypothyroidism with precocious puberty.

Unfortunately, the FSH and LH values are not usually helpful in the differential diagnosis between an ovarian tumor (pseudoprecocity) and idiopathic or CNS causes of true precocity. Distinguishing between low and normal values is difficult since there is considerable variation in levels throughout a 24-hour period. Furthermore, low levels are often found in the early stages of true precocity. In contrast, elevated LH values are suggestive of a gonadotropin-producing tumor or choriocarcinoma. The latter produces HCG, which cross-reacts with LH on the standard assay. In fact, most cases of choriocarcinoma can be diagnosed on the basis of a positive urine pregnancy test.

A vaginal smear or urocytogram confirms the presence of estrogenization. A typical smear in a patient with idiopathic precocious puberty might show 35 percent superficial, 50 percent intermediate, and 15 percent parabasal cells. The finding of estrogen excess (greater than 40 percent superficial cells) should raise the suspicion of an estrogen-secreting granulosa cell tumor. A high percentage of intermediate cells (95–100 percent) is seen in the luteal (or secretory)

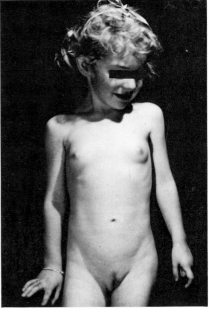

A

B

GROWTH CURVES OF WEIGHT BY AGE FOR GIRLS

(Average, Accelerated, and Retarded Rates of Maturation)

Case No. **PRECOCIOUS PUBERTY**

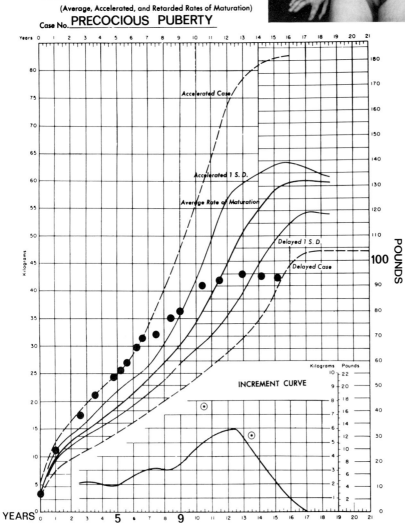

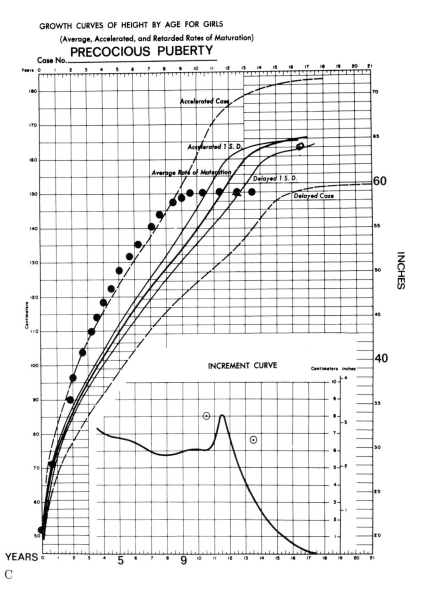

GROWTH CURVES OF HEIGHT BY AGE FOR GIRLS

(Average, Accelerated, and Retarded Rates of Maturation)

PRECOCIOUS PUBERTY

C

Fig. 5-1. Photograph of B.S. at age 3½. She was first brought to the clinic at age 3 years, 2 months for evaluation of "early development." Laboratory values included 17-ketosteroids, 1.8 mg/24 hours; a positive 24-hour urine test at 5 mouse units of FSH, and negative skull x-rays. Neurological exam was normal. B.S.'s menarche occurred at age 5½, and she attained adult height at age 10. Diagnosis was idiopathic precocious puberty. (A) Photograph, (B) weight chart, (C) height chart. (Reproduced from N. Bayley. Growth curves of height and weight by age for boys and girls, scaled according to physical maturity. J. Pediatr. 48:187, 1956. By permission of the author and the C. V. Mosby Co.)

phase of the normal ovulatory cycle and with progesterone-secreting thecomas. Clearly the date of the last menstrual period must be known to evaluate a vaginal smear. If an ovarian tumor is suspected, serum estradiol and progesterone levels should be measured. Estradiol levels are elevated in approximately one-third of patients with granulosa cell tumors. Serum progesterone and urinary pregnanediol are increased in the luteal phase of isosexual precocity and with ovarian thecomas. Laparoscopy is occasionally necessary, but it should be remembered that only about five percent of cases of sexual precocity are caused by ovarian tumors, and most of these are easily palpable.

Skull x-ray films, tomograms of the sella, and an EEG are indicated as initial screening tests. As it becomes more widely available, computerized axial tomography (CAT scan) may offer a noninvasive means of ruling out a CNS lesion. Invasive studies such as the pneumoencephalogram and cavernous sinogram should be done only on the basis of neurological signs and symptoms.

TREATMENT AND FOLLOW-UP

Treatment and follow-up depend on the diagnosis. Ovarian tumors and cysts should be surgically removed. Successful treatment of a tumor can be monitored by demonstrating decreasing estrogenization on vaginal smear and cessation of menses or by serum or urine estrogen levels, if available. Although in some patients excision of an ovarian cyst may result in regression of puberty, development sometimes continues, suggesting that the cyst was secondary to idiopathic precocious puberty and was not the primary etiology. Hypothalamic tumors and choriocarcinomas rarely are successfully treated surgically.

Precocity of the idiopathic or cerebral variety can be treated with medroxyprogesterone acetate (Depo-Provera), 150 mg intramuscularly every other week for two to four years or until age 8. Although such therapy results in cessation of menses and regression of breast development, the accelerated rate of bone maturation and the ultimate height are unchanged. Since the side effects are often considerable—excessive weight gain, rounded plethoric facies, hirsutism, and hypertension (all suggestive of glucocorticoid excess)—it may be better to avoid treating the child who has her menarche between 6 and 8 years of age [6]. Cyproterone acetate, an experimental drug with anti-androgenic properties, has been tried with variable results in patients with sexual precocity [7]. It is hoped that in the future specific anti-gonadotropin therapy will offer an effective alternative approach.

Despite the diagnosis of idiopathic precocious puberty, follow-up must continue at least every six months to exclude the possibility of organic disease not originally evident. Neurological status should be assessed by history and physical examination. Progress of pubertal development should be carefully recorded. Skull x-ray films, visual field exam (if practical), x-ray films for bone age, and perhaps an EEG are indicated annually.

It should be remembered that children with sexual precocity do not automatically manifest intellectual or psychosocial precocity. In fact, the degree of psychological maturity of a young girl is more likely to be related to the life experiences she encounters and transacts, her peer group, parent-child interactions, and sibling relationships. Parents tend to have abnormal expectations and fears for sexually precocious children in spite of the fact that psychologically such patients are more akin to children their own chronological age. Of utmost importance is the need to tell the young girl explicitly that her breast development is "early" but not "abnormal"; otherwise, she will conceive of herself as "freakish." In addition, it is important to tell the sexually precocious girl about menarche before its occurrence and to make sure that the school nurse has pads available. Psychological consultation for the family is often indicated to help them through this major stress [8].

HETEROSEXUAL PRECOCIOUS PUBERTY

Heterosexual precocity implies excess androgen production from an adrenal or ovarian source leading to acne, hirsutism, and virilization. The differential diagnosis includes (1) congenital adrenocortical hyperplasia (CAH), (2) adrenal tumors, and (3) ovarian tumors—arrhenoblastomas, lipoid cell, and Sertoli cell tumors.

PATIENT EVALUATION

The patient should be given a careful physical examination, especially noting evidence of hirsutism or clitoral enlargement and an adequate pelvic examination to exclude an ovarian mass. Ovarian tumors are usually palpable.

Laboratory tests include those mentioned for isosexual precocious puberty. In addition, a 24-hour urine test should be done for pregnanetriol, and if possible serum should be tested for 17-hydroxyprogesterone, dehydroepiandrosterone (DHA), DHA-sulfate (DHAS), 11-deoxycortisol, androstenedione, and testosterone. (See p. 27 for the pathways of steroid biosynthesis.) Urinary 17-ketosteroids and serum testosterone levels may help to distinguish between an adrenal and an ovarian source for the excess androgens. A normal urinary 17-ketosteroid level and an increased serum testosterone suggest an ovarian tumor. An elevated 17-ketosteroid level suppressible by dexamethasone is typical of CAH; this diagnosis can be confirmed by the finding of an elevated urinary pregnanetriol and increased serum 17-hydroxyprogesterone. An elevated 17-ketosteroid level not suppressible with dexamethasone is indicative of an adrenal or ovarian tumor. This differential diagnosis is made by intravenous pyelogram, pelvic examination under anesthesia, adrenal angiography and, if necessary, laparotomy.

TREATMENT AND FOLLOW-UP

Ovarian and adrenal tumors should be surgically excised, if possible. Patients with CAH should receive glucocorticoid replacement (e.g., hydrocortisone, 13–25 mg/M²/day divided into three daily dosages). Urinary 17-ketosteroids and growth should be monitored every three months. If the bone age is not too advanced, breast development may regress.

PREMATURE THELARCHE

Premature thelarche is defined as bilateral breast development without any other sign of puberty and is most commonly seen among young girls 1½ to 4 years of age. Occasionally, neonatal breast hypertrophy (secondary to fetal-placental estrogen) fails to regress within six months after birth; this persistent breast development is also characterized as premature thelarche. The typical child with premature thelarche has bilateral breast buds of 2–4 cm with little or no change in the nipple or areola. The breast tissue feels granular and may be slightly tender. In some cases, development is quite asymmetrical; one side may develop 6–12 months before the other. Growth is not accelerated, and the bone age is normal for height age. No other evidence of puberty appears; the labia remain prepubertal without obvious evidence of estrogen effect.

A vaginal smear or urocytogram may be atrophic or may show slight evidence of estrogen. In Grumbach's series [9] of patients with premature thelarche, 8 out of 9 patients showed 5 percent or greater superficial cells, but only 3 showed greater than 10 percent. Silver [10] demonstrated a slight estrogen effect in 15 out of 16 girls with premature thelarche as opposed to 7 out of 86 controls. In contrast to patients with isosexual precocity or normal puberty, the patient with premature thelarche still has a high percentage of parabasal cells. For example, a typical smear may show 7 percent superficial, 30 percent intermediate, and 63 percent parabasal and nonnucleated cells [11]. In addition, the evidence of estrogen effect on a vaginal smear or urocytogram is often transient. Similarly, estradiol levels (not necessary for the diagnosis) are also elevated in some patients [12].

Although the etiology of premature thelarche was originally thought to be increased end-organ sensitivity to low levels of endogenous estrogen, the evidence of at least transiently elevated estrogen levels suggests that small luteinized or cystic graafian follicles may be responsible for some cases. The waning of estrogen as the follicles become atretic would then correlate with the usual clinical course of regression or at least lack of progression of breast development.

PATIENT EVALUATION

The evaluation of a patient with premature breast development includes a careful review of medications and creams recently used. Occasionally it is discovered that a package of the mother's or sister's oral contraceptive pills has been ingested by the child. Premarin cream applied to the vulva nightly for more than two to three weeks may result in breast changes.

The physical examination should include notation of the appearance of the vaginal mucosa, size of the breasts, and a rectal examination to exclude an ovarian cyst. The uterus should not be enlarged in patients with premature thelarche. Growth charts, brought up to date, should indicate that the patient is continuing along her previously established percentile of height and weight. Laboratory tests include a skull x-ray film, vaginal smear or urocytogram for estrogen, and hand and wrist x-ray films for bone age.

TREATMENT AND FOLLOW-UP

Treatment consists mainly of reassurance and careful follow-up to confirm that the breast development does not represent the first sign of precocious puberty. A thorough physical examination should be done at each visit to detect a possible ovarian cyst. Height and bone age should be followed. Biopsy of the breast tissue is not indicated because removal of the breast bud prevents future normal development. In many cases, breast development does regress with age. Capraro's series of ten cases [13], followed 11 months to two years, showed four patients with no change in breast size, two with decreased breast size, one with regression after excision of luteinized follicle cysts, one with complete disappearance of breast development, and two lost to follow-up. Mothers should be reassured that pubertal development will occur at the normal adolescent age.

PREMATURE ADRENARCHE

Premature adrenarche is defined as the isolated appearance of pubic and occasionally axillary hair before the age of 8 without evidence of estrogenization or virilization. Most patients have a slight increase in urinary 17-ketosteroid production and increased plasma DHA and DHAS, suggesting that hormone biosynthesis in the adrenal gland undergoes maturation prematurely to a pubertal pattern [13]. Although production of these androgens is suppressible by dexamethasone and therefore dependent on adrenocorticotropic hormone, the mediator for the change at puberty and in premature adrenarche is unknown. Urinary 17-ketosteroids are elevated for chronological age, but they correspond with the levels expected for the amount of pubic hair (1–3 mg in 24 hours in most patients, occasionally up to 5 mg in 24 hours) [14, 15]. Bone age is usually normal or just slightly ad-

vanced. The vaginal smear is similar to that seen in normal prepubertal girls, e.g., 3 percent superficial, 17 percent intermediate, and
80 percent parabasal and nonnucleated cells [11].

The term *precocious pubarche* has been used by some authors to
denote the occasional patient with normal urinary 17-ketosteroids and
bone age who appears to have increased end-organ sensitivity to
circulating adrenal androgens. Other authors use the terms *adrenarche*
and *pubarche* synonymously.

PATIENT EVALUATION

The evaluation of the patient with premature adrenarche is similar
to that for heterosexual precocious puberty. The important findings
are the presence of pubic hair and the absence of breast development
or estrogenization of the labia and vagina. Virilization should not be
present.

The laboratory tests include an x-ray film of the wrist for bone age,
vaginal smear, and a 24-hour urine test for 17-ketosteroids. The differential diagnosis must exclude early precocious puberty, CAH, and an
adrenal or ovarian tumor. Sometimes the diagnosis of adrenarche is
made only in retrospect when further evidence of precocious puberty
does not occur. It should be recalled, however, that most patients with
precocious puberty have an advanced bone age, growth spurt, and
evidence of estrogenization on vaginal smear. Patients with CAH or
tumors usually have evidence of virilization (clitoral hypertrophy and
perhaps some fusion of the labia).

TREATMENT AND FOLLOW-UP

Treatment of premature adrenarche is reassurance and follow-up. The
child should be examined every 6 months to confirm the original diagnostic impression; evidence of virilization or early estrogen effect
imply a different diagnosis. Growth data should be carefully plotted,
and urinary 17-ketosteroid levels should be measured every 6–12
months. In general, pubertal development at adolescence can be
expected to be normal.

REFERENCES

1. Liu, N., et al.   Prevalence of EEG abnormalities in idiopathic precocious
   puberty and premature pubarche. *J. Clin. Endocrinol. Metab.* 25:1296,
   1965.
2. Sigurjonsdottir, T. J., and Hayles, A. B.   Precocious puberty: A report
   of 96 cases. *Am. J. Dis. Child.* 115:309, 1968.
3. Thamdrup, E.   Precocious sexual development. *Dan. Med. Bull.* 8:140,
   1961.
4. Cloutier, M. D., and Hayles, A. B.   Precocious puberty. *Adv. Pediatr.*
   17:125, 1970.
5. Ross, G., and Vande Wiele, R.   The Ovaries. In Williams, R. (Ed.),
   Textbook of Endocrinology (5th ed.). Philadelphia: Saunders, 1974.

6. Richman, R., et al. Adverse effects of large doses of MPA in idiopathic isosexual precocity. *J. Pediatr.* 79:963, 1971.
7. Bierich, J. Sexual precocity. *Clin. Endocrinol. Metabol.* 4(1):107, 1975.
8. Hampton, J. G., and Money, J. Idiopathic sexual precocity in the female. *Psychosom. Med.* 17:16, 1955.
9. Collett-Solberg, P., and Grumbach, M. A simplified procedure for evaluating estrogenic effects and the sex chromatin pattern in exfoliated cells in urine. *J. Pediatr.* 66:883, 1965.
10. Silver, H. K., and Sarni, D. Premature thelarche. *Pediatrics* 34:107, 1964.
11. Lencioni, L. H., and Staffieri, J. J. Urocytogram diagnosis of sexual precocity. *Acta Cytol.* (Baltimore) 13:382, 1969.
12. Jenner, M. R., et al. Hormonal changes in puberty: Plasma estradiol, LH, and FSH in prepubertal children, pubertal females, and in precocious puberty, premature thelarche, hypogonadism, and in a child with a feminizing ovarian tumor. *J. Clin. Endocrinol. Metab.* 34:521, 1972.
13. Capraro, V., et al. Premature thelarche. *Obstet. Gynecol. Surv.* 26:2, 1971.
14. Rosenfield, R. Plasma 17-ketosteroids and 17 β-hydroxysteroids in girls with premature development of sexual hair. *J. Pediatr.* 79:260, 1971.
15. Sigurjonsdottir, T. J., and Hayles, A. B. Premature pubarche. *Clin. Pediatr.* (Phila.) 7:29, 1968.

6. Menstrual Irregularities

This chapter presents a simplified approach to patients with delayed sexual development, amenorrhea, and dysfunctional uterine bleeding. Chapters 1 and 4 should be mastered before an evaluation of any of these problems is undertaken. Embryogenesis is reviewed in Chapter 2. The goal of such a workup should be to rule out a tumor or systemic disease and to make as exact a diagnosis as possible in order to present a discussion and treatment plan to the teenage girl and her parents.

The six sections in this chapter outline a program for evaluating the common developmental and menstrual problems of adolescence: (1) delayed sexual development, (2) delayed menarche with some pubertal development, (3) delayed menarche plus virilization, (4) secondary amenorrhea, (5) oligomenorrhea, and (6) dysfunctional uterine bleeding. The etiologies for different problems clearly overlap, and therefore the reader is sometimes referred back to an earlier section for definition and treatment. For example, the patient with XX/XO (Turner's mosaic) may present with delayed pubertal development, delayed menarche, or secondary amenorrhea. To prevent repetition, the discussion of this syndrome is found only in the section on delayed sexual development. Several illustrative case histories are included at the end of each of the first four sections.

A careful history and physical examination are mandatory whenever the patient expresses concern about her development or menstrual periods. Criteria for the physician to initiate a thorough workup are given in each section. The pertinent past history should include:

1. Neonatal history: maternal ingestion of hormones (e.g., Pranone,* Norlutin) that cause virilization; lymphedema (Turner's syndrome); previous miscarriages.
2. Family history: heights of all family members; age of menarche and fertility of sisters, mother, grandmothers, and aunts. (Familial disorders include delayed menarche, testicular feminization, congenital adrenal hyperplasia, and chromatin positive gonadal dysgenesis.)
3. Previous surgery, irradiation, or chemotherapy.
4. Review of systems with special emphasis on a recent history of abdominal pain, diarrhea, headaches, weight changes, or emotional stresses.
5. Age of initiation of pubertal development, if any, and rate of development.

* Pranone is no longer used commercially.

6. Growth data plotted on charts, such as those illustrated in Chapter 4. No growth for several years may suggest a chronic disease such as Crohn's disease or an acquired endocrine disorder.

The appropriate diagnostic tests are thus dictated by the clinical situation and the findings on the initial physical examination.

DELAYED SEXUAL DEVELOPMENT

If there is no evidence of breast budding or pubic hair by the age of 14 and certainly by age 15, a careful evaluation is required. The stigmata of Turner's syndrome, especially short stature, may prompt an earlier diagnosis. A patient history and physical examination are essential. The chief complaint may be "no development," and yet evidence of breast budding and a growth spurt often exclude this diagnosis. Although a speculum examination of the vagina is crucial in the evaluation of the patient with delayed menarche (see the section on delayed menarche with some pubertal development), visualizing the cervix in the patient with no sexual development is much less essential in the initial workup. However, in the nonobese prepubertal teenager, a simple bimanual rectal-abdominal exam will often allow palpation of the cervix and sometimes the uterus.

The history, physical examination, and growth data will often determine the laboratory tests necessary for the workup of the female with sexual infantilism. The tests may include a complete blood count (CBC), sedimentation rate, thyroxine (T_4), resin-triiodothyronine (RT_3), skull x-ray films, bone age, buccal smear, and levels of follicle-stimulating hormone (FSH) and luteinizing hormone (LH). Hypothyroidism, Crohn's disease, and anorexia nervosa should be evident before gonadotropin levels are drawn. The differential diagnosis is simplified by separating patients into categories on the basis of FSH and LH levels. As mentioned in Chapter 4, serum for FSH and LH can be sent by the primary care physician to the endocrine laboratory of a teaching hospital or a reliable commercial laboratory. High FSH and LH levels imply ovarian failure. Low or normal levels of FSH and LH imply a central nervous system (CNS) etiology—CNS tumor, hypopituitarism, hypothalamic dysfunction—or a systemic disease (Fig. 6-1).

High Follicle-Stimulating and Luteinizing Hormone Levels

Gonadal dysgenesis

Slightly over one-half of patients with gonadal dysgenesis are XO (Turner's syndrome). The classic stigmata of Turner's syndrome include short stature (final height less than 58 inches), widely spaced nipples, webbed neck, low hairline, short fourth and/or fifth meta-

73

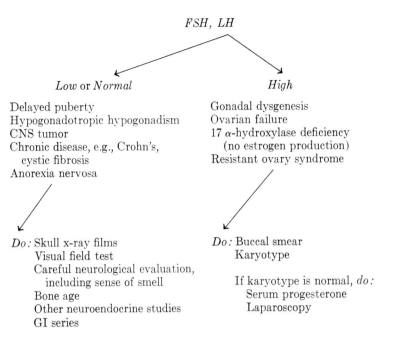

FSH, LH

Low or Normal   High

Delayed puberty   Gonadal dysgenesis
Hypogonadotropic hypogonadism   Ovarian failure
CNS tumor   17 α-hydroxylase deficiency
Chronic disease, e.g., Crohn's,   (no estrogen production)
  cystic fibrosis   Resistant ovary syndrome
Anorexia nervosa

Do: Skull x-ray films   Do: Buccal smear
    Visual field test   Karyotype
    Careful neurological evaluation,
      including sense of smell   If karyotype is normal, do:
    Bone age   Serum progesterone
    Other neuroendocrine studies   Laparoscopy
    GI series

Fig. 6-1. Differential diagnosis of delayed development.

carpals, cubitus valgus, ptosis, low-set ears, narrow, high-arched palate, and multiple pigmented nevi. Associated problems include cardiac anomalies (especially coarctation of the aorta), renal anomalies, otitis media, and mastoiditis, and an increased incidence of hypertension, achlorhydria, diabetes mellitus, and Hashimoto's thyroiditis [1, 2]. A young adolescent with Turner's syndrome has prepubertal female genitalia, bilateral streak gonads, and a normal uterus and vagina capable of responding to exogenous hormones. An older adolescent (over 15 or 16 years old) with undiagnosed or untreated Turner's syndrome typically has pubic and axillary hair (secondary to adrenal androgens) but no breast development or estrogenization of the vaginal mucosa (no ovarian function). Indeed, estrogenization in a patient with XO should raise the possibility of a theca lutein cyst or germ cell tumor.

The other 40–50 percent of patients with gonadal dysgenesis have a mosaic karyotype (e.g., XX/XO) or a structural abnormality of the second X chromosome (e.g., X-isoX). Such patients may show none or all of the classic stigmata of Turner's syndrome. Patients with Turner's mosaic may present with (1) sexual infantilism, (2) some sexual development and primary amenorrhea, (3) secondary amenorrhea and short stature, or (4) regular menses and normal stature. Gonadal failure is indicated by elevated gonadotropin levels. Rare pregnancies have been reported in patients with functioning gonads.

The term *pure gonadal dysgenesis* includes patients with normal or tall stature and the gonadal abnormality of Turner's syndrome. Breast development is absent or poor; gonadotropins are high. Proportions are usually eunuchoid. Karyotypes usually show mosaicism but may show XX or XY.

Patients with Turner's syndrome should not be treated with exogenous hormones until the age of 14 or 15 to allow maximal linear growth before the epiphyses are closed. The use of androgens is controversial and probably does not increase ultimate height. Our mode of therapy is to introduce conjugated estrogens (Premarin) at low dosage, 0.3 mg once daily, for approximately one year or until linear growth appears to be leveling off. The dosage is then increased to 0.625 mg given on days 1–21 of each month, with 10 mg of medroxy-progesterone (Provera) added on days 17–21 to give cyclic withdrawal bleeding.* Increasing the Premarin dosage to 1.25–2.5 mg on days 1–21 may improve breast development and may be required for normal menstruation.

Patients with gonadal dysgenesis need an opportunity to express their feelings about their lack of development and short stature and to assimilate the long-range problem of infertility. Denial of the diagnosis between visits is common and the same questions may arise each time. There is some evidence that patients cope better with the issue of infertility if they receive such information in response to their own questions rather than as part of a didactic lecture gratuitously given by the doctor [4]. Not infrequently, a young patient will request to be excused from physical education classes so that her lack of development will not be the subject of peer discussion; this request should be honored. Emphasis should be placed on the ability of the young woman to be a normal wife and the mother of adopted children.

In the rare case of a patient with an XY line in the karyotype (mixed gonadal dysgenesis [see page 87] removal of the gonads is required because of the malignant potential.

Ovarian failure

A past history of a malignancy treated with irradiation (greater than 1500 rads to the pelvis) and chemotherapy (e.g., cyclophosphamide) suggest the diagnosis of ovarian failure. In unexplained cases of ovarian failure, laparoscopy is indicated. Treatment is identical with that for gonadal dysgenesis.

---

* Although an increased risk of endometrial carcinoma has been reported in postmenopausal women taking conjugated estrogen [3], no such association has been reported thus far for the cyclic use of conjugated estrogen and medroxyprogesterone in patients with ovarian failure, perhaps because the addition of progesterone induces withdrawal flow and prevents endometrial hyperplasia.

17 α-Hydroxylase deficiency

17 α-Hydroxylase deficiency, an extremely rare disorder, is associated with adrenal insufficiency and hypertension. Gonadotropins are elevated because the ovary fails to secrete estrogen. Plasma progesterone is elevated.

Resistant ovary syndrome

In resistant ovary syndrome, a rare condition, the ovaries appear normal at laparoscopy. Biopsy reveals numerous primordial follicles. Presumably the ovaries lack a receptor site for gonadotropin function. A trial of exogenous human gonadotropins is indicated to exclude the remote possibility that the patient has an abnormally structured FSH and LH.

NORMAL OR LOW FOLLICLE-STIMULATING AND LUTEINIZING HORMONE LEVELS

Delayed puberty versus hypogonadotropic hypogonadism

The diagnosis of delayed puberty is made by excluding an organic cause. If symptoms of a functional disorder (e.g., anorexia nervosa, depression) or a chronic disease (e.g., Crohn's disease) are absent, a neurological evaluation and neuroendocrine studies are required to rule out a hypothalamic or pituitary lesion. Studies may include skull x-ray films, electroencephalogram (EEG), growth hormone levels, metyrapone test, LH releasing hormone (LHRH) test (available in teaching centers), brain scan, computerized axial tomography (CAT scan), if available, and possibly a pneumoencephalogram. Neurological evaluation may reveal anosmia or other cranial nerve defects associated with hypogonadotropic hypogonadism. It should be mentioned that the term *hypogonadotropic hypogonadism* probably includes a diverse group of patients—some with LH releasing factor deficiency and some with gonadotropin (LH and/or FSH) deficiency. Gonadotropin deficiency may occur as an isolated problem or as part of panhypopituitarism with deficiencies of adrenocorticotropic hormone, thyroid-stimulating hormone, and growth hormone. Hypogonadotropic hypogonadism is also associated with the Laurence-Moon-Biedl and Prader-Willi syndromes.

If no secondary sexual development has occurred by the age of 15 or 16 and a tumor is not evident, the patient should probably receive substitution treatment similar to that used in patients with gonadal dysgenesis to induce sexual development. To delay therapy until a patient is 20 or 21 years old may do irreversible psychological harm. Patients with delayed puberty will eventually have pituitary function and may continue cycling, either spontaneously or with clomiphene citrate. Patients with hypogonadotropism will require prolonged substitution therapy with estrogens and progesterone; human gonado-tropins, and perhaps in the future LHRH, may be used to induce ovulation in patients desiring fertility.

Central nervous system tumor

A CNS tumor is a rare cause of sexual infantilism. Skull films may show an enlarging sella; visual fields may be constricted. It should be noted, however, that even though a CNS tumor is not obvious at the time of the initial workup, it may become evident several years later when skull x-ray films suddenly demonstrate an enlarging sella or the patient begins to complain of headaches or vomiting. Reevaluation every six months is necessary for a suspected but unconfirmed lesion. Invasive studies such as the pneumoencephalogram and cavernous sinogram should be undertaken if suspicion of a tumor is strong.

Most patients with CNS tumors require substitution therapy with estrogen and progesterone to induce breast development and menstrual periods. Because of the frequently associated adrenal insufficiency, pubic and axillary hair may remain scanty or absent.

Crohn's disease

Delayed pubertal development may be the presenting complaint of some patients with regional enteritis. Occasionally the gastrointestinal history is negative; however, most patients have experienced inter-mittent crampy abdominal pain and either diarrhea or constipation. Typically the growth curve will show a leveling off of height and usually loss of weight. In most cases, the sedimentation rate is elevated and the hematocrit and albumin are low. If the etiology of delayed puberty remains in doubt, an upper gastrointestinal series with small bowel follow-through, a barium enema, and proctoscopy should be performed.

Anorexia nervosa

Patients with malnutrition and anorexia nervosa may have delayed development because of the failure to attain a critical body weight necessary for initiation of the hypothalamic-ovarian interaction (see reference 4 in Chap. 4). More commonly anorexia nervosa is a cause of secondary amenorrhea.

Case 1. S. T. presented to the clinic at age 15 with "no development." She had always been the shortest member of her class. The review of systems was unremarkable. Physical examination (Fig. 6-2) revealed a short teenager with many of the stigmata of Turner's syndrome (low hairline, webbed neck, ptosis, "fishmouth," increased carrying angle, and short fourth metacarpals). Her height was 54 inches and her weight, 105 pounds; blood pressure was 125/80; and pulse was 78. Breast development was stage I, and no pubic or axillary hair was present.

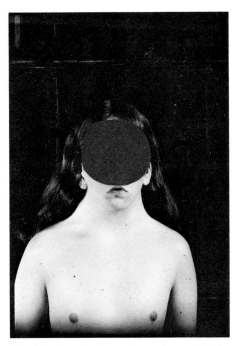

Fig. 6-2. Case 1: Turner's syndrome (XO).

Pertinent laboratory tests showed an FSH 143 mIU/ml, LH 135 mIU/ml, a chromatin negative buccal smear, and karyotype of XO. The patient was started on conjugated estrogens and then was cycled after one year with medroxyprogesterone.

Case 2. C. O. was referred to our unit at age $15^{10}/_{12}$ for delayed development. She was the 7 pound, 6 ounce product of a normal pregnancy and delivery. Her developmental milestones were normal; however, she was always the shortest member of her class (she was an A student in the tenth grade). The review of systems was negative. The family history revealed that one of her father's sisters had her menarche at age 20. On physical examination (Fig. 6-3) C.O. was a short, pleasant teenager with a height of $55\frac{3}{4}$ inches and a weight of 86 pounds; blood pressure was 105/70; pulse was 66. Fundi were normal. Breast development was stage I, although the areolae were slightly puffy with a diameter of 2.4 cm. There was no pubic or axillary hair. As an outpatient, C.O. had a normal CBC, blood urea nitrogen, thyroid function tests, and urinalysis; FSH was 7.7 mIU/ml and LH 6.3 mIU/ml. She was admitted for an extensive neuroendocrine evaluation, which included normal skull x-ray films, EEG, CAT scan, metyrapone test, growth hormone levels, LHRH test, and visual field exam.

Because no organic lesion was found, the patient was started on conjugated estrogens (Premarin) 0.3 mg daily, and within a short period of time she began to have breast development. Pubic hair appeared gradually. One year later the Premarin dosage was increased to 0.625 mg on days 1–21 each month and Provera 10 mg was added on days 17–21. A trial period without

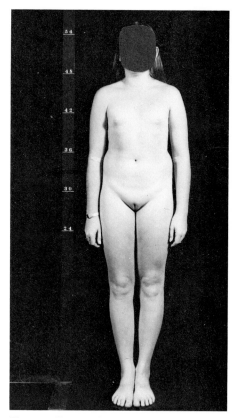

Fig. 6-3. Case 2: delayed puberty.

hormones is planned in the future. At the present time, C.O.'s diagnosis remains in doubt—delayed puberty versus hypogonadotropic hypogonadism. In addition to the hormone treatment, she will continue to receive careful neurological follow-up to exclude an unsuspected CNS lesion.

DELAYED MENARCHE WITH SOME PUBERTAL DEVELOPMENT

In considering the evaluation of the young woman with delayed menarche (no periods by age 16) or primary amenorrhea (no periods by age 18), the physician needs to know the range of normal (see Chap. 4) and the patient's previous development. If a young woman presents for evaluation at age 15 and history reveals that her pubertal development began at age 14, one can usually reassure her that she can expect her menarche by age 16 or 17. Documentation of steady progression of sexual development and growth and a careful explanation to the patient of the variability in development are essential. A patient who has not had her menarche by age 16 and yet started her

Hypothalamus	Familial
	Stress
	Anorexia nervosa
	Obesity
	Drugs (e.g., pheno-thiazines)
Pituitary	Idiopathic hypopitui-tarism
	Tumor
Adrenal	CAH (mild deficiency of 3 β-hydroxy-steroid dehydro-genase or 17 α-hy-droxylase)
Ovary	Gonadal dysgenesis
	Ovarian failure
	Stein-Leventhal syn-drome
	Tumor
Uterus	Agenesis
	Testicular feminiza-tion
Vagina	Imperforate hymen
	Agenesis

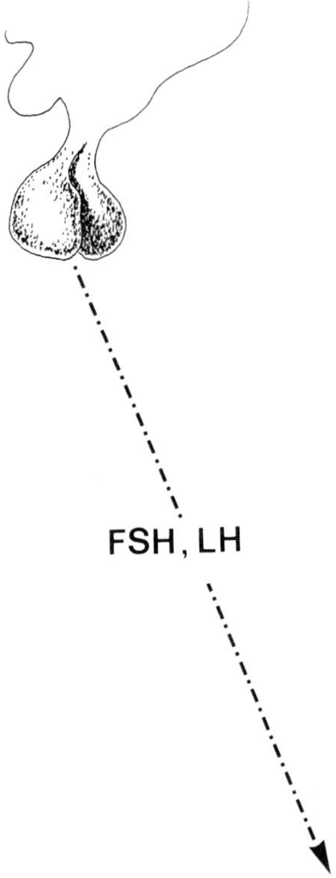

FSH, LH

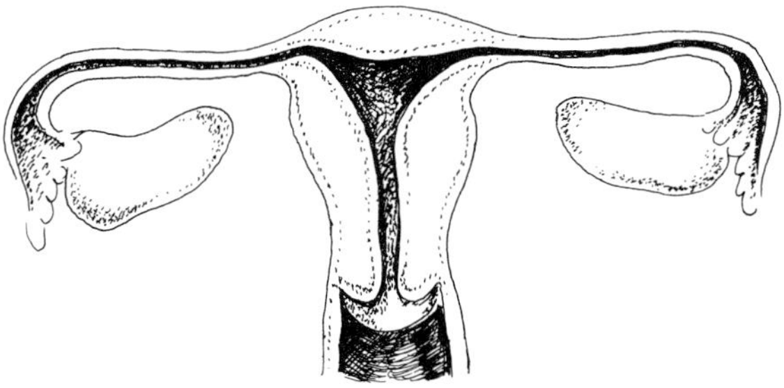

Fig. 6-4. Etiology of primary amenorrhea.

development at age 12 requires a thorough evaluation for cause. The causes of amenorrhea should be considered in terms of anatomical etiologies (Fig. 6-4). These categories should help direct the physician to the necessary laboratory tests.

A careful physical examination gives an excellent indication of the endogenous hormone levels. It should be recalled that adrenal androgens are largely responsible for pubic and axillary hair; estrogen is responsible for breast development, menses, and maturation of the external genitalia, vagina, and uterus.

Unlike the patient who presents with no sexual development, the patient with no menses must be carefully examined to rule out an external or internal genital anomaly. If the examination is normal, assessment of estrogen effect allows the physician to divide the patients into two main categories, as indicated in Figure 6-5. The most important features of the evaluation are the physical examination, response to intramuscular progesterone, gonadotropin levels, and if necessary a buccal smear (and/or karyotype).

WITHDRAWAL BLEEDING AFTER INTRAMUSCULAR PROGESTERONE

Delayed menarche (with adequate estrogen and normal anatomy)

In most cases, the teenager is healthy and will eventually begin spontaneous periods. Factors such as weight [5] (either too little or too much), stress, and depression appear to act at the hypothalamic level to prevent the onset of normal cycles. An adequate workup consists of a careful physical examination, vaginal smear positive for estrogen, withdrawal bleeding to intramuscular progesterone, hemoglobin, and urinalysis. Thyroid disease and diabetes mellitus should be excluded by physical examination and/or laboratory tests (glucose, T_4, RT_3).

If by age 16 to 18 the young woman desires normal periods, she can be cycled with Provera, 10 mg for five days every six to twelve weeks. This medication will produce a secretory endometrium and withdrawal periods. Moreover, the drug may prevent endometrial hyperplasia from unopposed estrogen stimulation. Withdrawal flow also confirms the continuing presence of circulating endogenous estrogens and indirectly a functioning pituitary gland.

For the woman older than 18, clomiphene citrate, a drug that acts at the hypothalamic level to stimulate the release of LH releasing factor and thereby FSH and LH, may be prescribed by the gynecologist to confirm the presence of an intact hypothalamic-ovarian axis. A period is produced with intramuscular progesterone, and then clomiphene citrate is given 50 mg daily for five days starting on day 5 of the period. Basal body temperatures are monitored to see if ovulation occurs. If the patient ovulates and has a normal period, clomiphene can be continued for three months. If basal body charts show no evidence of ovulation, clomiphene can be increased to 100 mg daily for five days. Careful follow-up with repeat pelvic exams every month is essential to prevent hyperstimulation and cystic enlargement of the ovaries [6]. It should be noted that the hypothalamus does not become responsive to clomiphene until middle to late puberty. The advantage of the drug is that occasionally the patient may develop spontaneous menses following treatment; the disadvantage is that the sexually active teenager may become pregnant. Thus, it may seem wise to reserve this medication for use as a fertility drug.

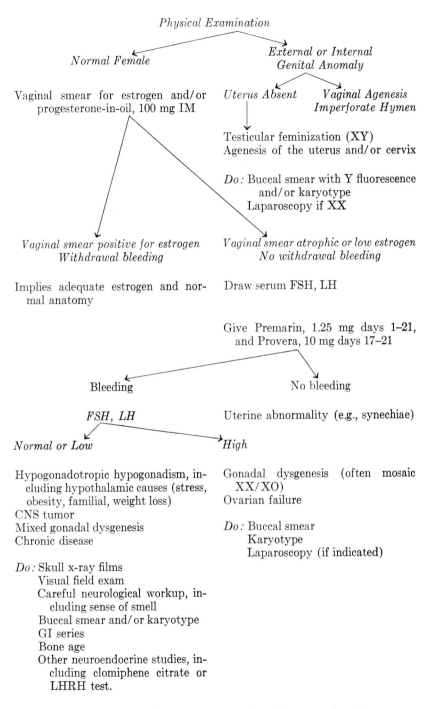

Physical Examination

Normal Female

External or Internal Genital Anomaly

Vaginal smear for estrogen and/or progesterone-in-oil, 100 mg IM

Uterus Absent

Vaginal Agenesis Imperforate Hymen

Testicular feminization (**XY**)
Agenesis of the uterus and/or cervix

Do: Buccal smear with Y fluorescence and/or karyotype
Laparoscopy if **XX**

Vaginal smear positive for estrogen Withdrawal bleeding

Vaginal smear atrophic or low estrogen No withdrawal bleeding

Implies adequate estrogen and normal anatomy

Draw serum FSH, LH

Give Premarin, 1.25 mg days 1–21, and Provera, 10 mg days 17–21

Bleeding

No bleeding

FSH, LH

Uterine abnormality (e.g., synechiae)

Normal or Low

High

Hypogonadotropic hypogonadism, including hypothalamic causes (stress, obesity, familial, weight loss)
CNS tumor
Mixed gonadal dysgenesis
Chronic disease

Do: Skull x-ray films
Visual field exam
Careful neurological workup, including sense of smell
Buccal smear and/or karyotype
GI series
Bone age
Other neuroendocrine studies, including clomiphene citrate or LHRH test.

Gonadal dysgenesis (often mosaic XX/XO)
Ovarian failure

Do: Buccal smear
Karyotype
Laparoscopy (if indicated)

Fig. 6-5. Workup of delayed menarche in females with some pubertal development.

No Withdrawal Bleeding After Intramuscular Progesterone

Low or normal follicle-stimulating and luteinizing hormone levels

HYPOGONADOTROPIC HYPOGONADISM

In contrast to the patients discussed on p. 75 with sexual infantilism, low levels of gonadotropins may induce some estrogen effect, scanty breast development, and slight maturation of the vaginal mucosa and labia. In some cases gonadotropin and estrogen levels appear to be normal at the onset of puberty and then diminish secondary to depression, stress, or weight loss. The same considerations in terms of excluding an organic lesion (e.g., CNS tumor, idiopathic hypopituitarism) or a systemic disease are applicable.

If possible, therapy should be directed at the underlying cause of hypogonadotropism. For example, weight loss secondary to depression should be treated with psychiatric and dietary counseling, not with hormones. However, if an organic lesion or emotional problem is excluded and the patient remains poorly estrogenized at age 16 or 17, development can be stimulated and menses produced with exogenous hormones: conjugated estrogens (Premarin), 0.625 or 1.25 mg, or ethinyl estradiol, 0.1 mg, on days 1–21 of each month, *plus* medroxyprogesterone (Provera), 10 mg on days 17–21. Therapy should be discontinued once a year for three months to reassess the patient's hypothalamic-pituitary-ovarian axis. Gonadotropin levels (FSH and LH) should be measured at the end of the three months. Some patients may begin spontaneous cycling. If infertility is a later problem, treatment with clomiphene or human gonadotropins is indicated. Patients with hypogonadotropism should be carefully followed by neurological examination, x-ray films of the sella, and visual field tests to rule out the presence of an underlying CNS tumor not evident on initial examination.

OTHER CONDITIONS

Other conditions occurring with low or normal FSH and LH levels are CNS tumor and Crohn's disease (see p. 76), and (rarely) mixed gonadal dysgenesis (see p. 87).

High follicle-stimulating and luteinizing hormone levels

Conditions occurring with high FSH and LH levels and no withdrawal bleeding after intramuscular progesterone are gonadal dysgenesis (see p. 72) and ovarian failure (see p. 74).

External or Internal Genital Anomalies

Vaginal agenesis and imperforate hymen

The diagnosis of imperforate hymen should be made by visual inspection long before the expected menarche. Referral to a sympathetic gynecologist is essential. Patients with vaginal agenesis usually have agenesis or anomalies of the uterus and commonly have skeletal and renal anomalies.

Testicular feminization

The patient with classic testicular feminization (male pseudohermaphroditism, or perhaps "gonadal dysgenesis with female sex assignment") has good breast development and absent or very sparse pubic and axillary hair. The vagina is short, and the uterus and cervix are absent. The chromosome pattern is XY. The gonads, which may be intraabdominal or in the inguinal rings, are testes; thus the blood testosterone level is in the range of the normal male. Because of insensitivity to androgens and enhanced estrogen production, the patient develops a female habitus and external genitalia. The lack of pubic and axillary hair is the result of end-organ failure to respond to adrenal and testicular androgens.

Because the testes in such patients have a high rate of malignant degeneration, they should be prophylactically removed after the patient has attained full height and breast development. After surgery, the patient should receive cyclic Premarin therapy, 0.625 mg daily on days 1–21 of each month.

Before surgery is undertaken, the patient needs to understand her anatomy. The physician should stress the patient's femininity and her ability to have normal sexual relations; she must, however, ultimately accept the fact that she cannot have menses or bear children. Relating the etiology to "genes" or "chromosomes" is more helpful than telling her that she is a "male" or "XY." If the question "Am I XY?" arises in the course of discussion, the physician needs to answer the question honestly and at the same time reemphasize that the patient's phenotype is female. The necessary laparotomy should be explained as removal of "gonads" rather than testes; gonads can be viewed as organs that did not develop into either testes or ovaries because of the "chromosome problem." The tumor risk can be openly discussed.

Partial testicular feminization has also been reported; the patient had an XY karyotype, labial fusion, a blind vas deferens, and testes located in the labioscrotal folds. At puberty, the patient developed breasts and pubic and axillary hair. Because of the absence of the uterus, the patient presented with amenorrhea[7].

Agenesis of the uterus and/or cervix

Patients with agenesis of the uterus and/or cervix appear as normal estrogenized females with pubic and axillary hair. Absence of the uterus is often associated with anomalies of the urinary tract. Laparoscopy should be done to rule out cervical atresia with an intact uterus [8]. No hormonal treatment is necessary if the patient has functioning ovaries.

Case 3. E. B. presented to the clinic at age 16 with a history of "no periods." Breast and pubic hair development had started at age 11 or 12. She had noted a slight whitish vaginal discharge for several years. On physical examination E. B. was a healthy, attractive teenage girl with a height of 64 inches and a weight of 125 pounds. Breast development was stage V, and pubic hair stage IV. Pelvic examination revealed a well-estrogenized vagina and a normal cervix and uterus. A vaginal smear showed 20 percent superficial and 80 percent intermediate cells. Following an intramuscular injection of 100 mg progesterone-in-oil, she had a four-day period. She began spontaneous menses two months later and has continued normal cycling.

Case 4. P. M. presented to the clinic at age 18 for evaluation of "no periods." She had breast development at age 13; however, she had not noted any development of pubic or axillary hair. She had recently gained 70 pounds, seemingly secondary to the anxiety over her lack of periods. On physical examination P. M. was an attractive, overweight young woman with a height of 64 inches and a weight of 187 pounds. Blood pressure was 140/80; pulse was 80. Breasts were stage V and pendulous. No axillary or pubic hair was present. Pelvic examination revealed a short vagina with no cervix or uterus. Laboratory tests showed a chromatin negative buccal smear with fluorescent Y bodies in 60 percent of the cells. Karyotype was XY. Urinary 17-hydroxy-corticosteroids were 7.7 mg/24 hours; 17-ketosteroids were 24 mg/24 hours. Serum testosterone was 281 ng/100 ml (the level for a normal female is up to 80 ng/100 ml). A diagnosis of testicular feminization syndrome (male pseudohermaphroditism) was made. After elective surgery to remove the intraabdominal testes, P. M. was started on conjugated estrogens (Premarin), 0.625 mg on days 1–21 of each month. She required extensive counseling concerning the issue of her femininity and her inability to bear children. She subsequently lost 35 pounds by dieting.

Case 5. R. L. presented to the clinic at age 18 for evaluation of "no periods." She recalled that her breast and pubic hair development had started at age 12. She had always been the shortest member of her class, and she had worn bilateral hearing aids since age 11. On physical examination (Fig. 6-6) R. L. was a short, overweight black female with a height of 51 inches and a weight of 105 pounds. She had hypertelorism, ptosis, a low hairline, an increased carrying angle, and short fourth metacarpals. Breast development was stage V; pubic hair was stage IV. Pelvic examination revealed a poorly estrogenized vagina with a small cervix and uterus. Vaginal smear showed no evidence of estrogen. Laboratory tests revealed a serum FSH of 258 mIU/ml and LH of 173 mIU/ml (indicative of ovarian failure). Karyotype was 46, X-isoX. The patient was cycled with conjugated estrogen (Premarin) and medroxyprogesterone (Provera) and had normal withdrawal flow each month.

DELAYED MENARCHE PLUS VIRILIZATION

In the rare situation of significant hirsutism and/or virilization associated with delayed menarche, additional studies are necessary to make the diagnosis. Laboratory tests may include a buccal smear

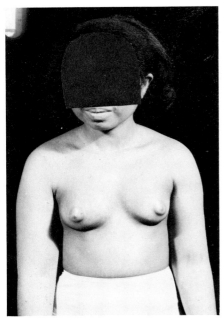

Fig. 6-6. Case 5: gonadal dysgenesis, karyotype 46, X-isoX.

(karyotype), 24-hour urine for 17-ketosteroids and 17-hydroxycorti-
costeroids, serum testosterone, FSH, and LH. Laparoscopy is often
indicated. The differential diagnosis includes (1) congenital adrenocortical hyperplasia, (2) ovarian and adrenal tumors, (3) Stein-
Leventhal syndrome, (4) mixed gonadal dysgenesis, (5) incomplete
form of testicular feminization, (6) gonadal dysgenesis (with virilization), and (7) true hermaphroditism.

Congenital Adrenocortical Hyperplasia

To pediatricians, the diagnosis of congenital adrenocortical hyperplasia (CAH) usually implies the virilized newborn with or without a
salt-losing tendency. Some patients, however, may have a mild block
of their adrenal steroid synthesis (11 β-hydroxylase or 21-hydroxylase
deficiency) and may therefore manifest clitoromegaly and subsequent
virilization with puberty. Patients may present with delayed menarche
or oligomenorrhea. Those with 11 β-hydroxylase deficiency may have
associated hypertension. The pathways of steroid biosynthesis are
shown in Figure 6-7; normal values for 17-ketosteroids are given in
Appendix 1. In patients with CAH, urinary 17-ketosteroids are
elevated and suppressible by dexamethasone, 0.5 mg orally every 6
hours for four days. Occasionally a two-week course of dexamethasone

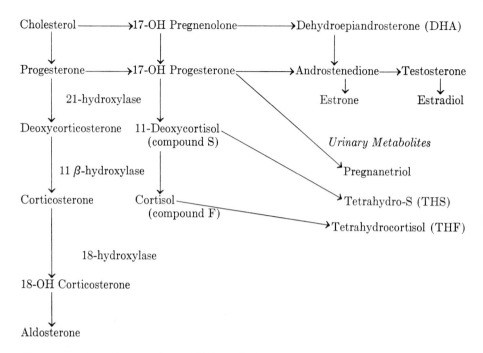

Fig. 6-7. Major pathways of steroid biosynthesis.

or a dose of 2 mg every 6 hours for three days is necessary for diagnostic suppression.

Treatment for CAH consists of glucocorticoid replacement. Prednisone, 5 mg in the morning and 2.5 mg in the evening, is usually sufficient, but the response must be determined by following urinary 17-ketosteroids and the subsequent course. In mild cases dexamethasone, 0.5 mg daily at bedtime, may be adequate therapy.

OVARIAN AND ADRENAL TUMORS

Patients may present with virilization from ovarian or adrenal tumors either before or after the onset of puberty or the menarche. Depending on the androgen produced, 17-ketosteroids may be elevated. If testosterone is the major hormone secreted, 17-ketosteroids may be in the normal range in spite of severe virilization. Patients with elevated 17-ketosteroids (usually greater than 25 mg/24 hours) will not show suppression with dexamethasone, 0.5–2 mg every 6 hours for four days. Treatment is usually surgical.

STEIN-LEVENTHAL SYNDROME

A discussion of the Stein-Leventhal syndrome can be found on pages 91 and 143. In rare cases the syndrome is responsible for delayed menarche with moderate virilization.

MIXED GONADAL DYSGENESIS

At puberty patients with mixed gonadal dysgenesis (MGD) show virilization (without evidence of estrogen effect) because the functioning intraabdominal testis produces testosterone. The chromosome patterns of patients with MGD include XY, XO/XY, XX/XY, XO/XX/XY, XO, and XO/XS. The gonadal constitution in Federman's series in *Abnormal Sexual Development* [7] consisted of:

Testis plus streak gonad	24 patients
Unilateral testis only	9 patients
Streak gonad plus tumor	7 patients
Testis plus tumor	1 patient
Unilateral tumor only	1 patient
	42 patients

All patients had a uterus. Because the dysgenetic intraabdominal testis has a high incidence of malignant transformation, it should be removed. Fertility is impossible. Patients can be given cyclic Premarin and Provera to produce menses.

INCOMPLETE FORM OF TESTICULAR FEMINIZATION

Patients with incomplete testicular feminization have an XY chromosomal pattern, agenesis of the uterus, hirsutism, clitoral enlargement, and absence of breast development. One family has been shown to have testicular 17-ketosteroid reductase deficiency; in another family possible 5 α-reductase deficiency may have prevented the conversion of testosterone to dihydrotestosterone and thus the differentiation of the urogenital sinus and urogenital tubercle into male external genitalia. Unlike classic testicular feminization (see pp. 24 and 83) which has enhanced estrogen production, the estrogen levels in these patients are low, and therefore breast development is absent at puberty. Treatment consists of surgical removal of the testes and replacement treatment with Premarin [9, 10, 11].

GONADAL DYSGENESIS (XO) WITH VIRILIZATION

Rarely, patients with gonadal dysgenesis may show virilization at puberty. The streak gonads may contain Leydig-like cells that presumably secrete androgens. Laparoscopy should rule out the possibility of a tumor. Mosaicism with a Y line should be excluded by karyotype and Y fluorescence of a buccal smear.

TRUE HERMAPHRODITISM

A true hermaphrodite is a patient with ovarian and testicular tissue. The majority of the patients are XX, although there are some mosaics including XX/XY (may be an overlap with MGD) and XX/XXY. Although the majority of patients are raised as males, a few appear as almost normal females with mild to moderate virilization at puberty, depending on the balance of ovarian and testicular function. Gonadotropins may be normal or high. The majority of patients with this rare diagnosis present in the newborn period with ambiguous genitalia.

Case 6. C. R. presented to the clinic at age 16 with a complaint of "no periods." She had noted increasing hair under her chin beginning at age 15, and she had gained 30–40 pounds in the previous year. On physical examination C. R. was an overweight, hirsute teenager with a height of 62 inches and a weight of 156 pounds. Blood pressure and pulse were normal. She had coarse hair over her face, neck, and back. Breast and pubic hair development were stage V. Pelvic examination revealed mild clitoromegaly, a normal cervix and uterus, and questionably enlarged ovaries. Urinary 17-ketosteroids were 7.7 mg/24 hours; serum testosterone was elevated at 239 ng/100 ml. At laparoscopy C. R. was found to have the enlarged polycystic ovaries of the Stein-Leventhal syndrome. She was placed on oral contraceptive pills, and serum testosterone fell to 34 ng/100 ml. She has had no further progression of her hirsutism.

SECONDARY AMENORRHEA

PATIENT EVALUATION

Many of the causes of delayed menarche are also responsible for secondary amenorrhea. The two most common causes of missed periods in the adolescent are pregnancy and stress. Because of the availability of abortion, a period that is two to three weeks overdue should be investigated at least to rule out pregnancy (see Chap. 1, p. 18 for a review of pregnancy tests). A history to the contrary should never be reassuring. Many older teenagers are still fearful of admitting a past history of intercourse; at age 11 or 12 a youngster may not understand her own anatomy well enough to answer the questions accurately. Excessive concern about a period two weeks late should prompt the physician to explore with the teenager a history of unprotected sexual relations.

Stress and changes in environment are responsible for most cases of missed periods in adolescents. Young women are especially likely to have irregular periods with fevers, emotional upset, weight changes, or changes in environment such as summer camp, boarding school, or college. Many patients with classic anorexia nervosa present to the physician for evaluation of secondary amenorrhea; frequently the magnitude of the weight loss is evident only after a careful history and weight charts from the pediatrician's office or school are obtained. Both parents and patient may initially deny any change in weight or emotional issues. Similarly, a patient with depression may rapidly gain weight and become amenorrheic. It is not uncommon to find the adolescent viewing the weight gain as secondary to the loss of periods and retention of blood. The patient with anorexia or depression requires counseling for emotional problems as well as reassurance about the eventual return of her cycles.

Teenagers often have irregular periods with amenorrhea for six to twelve months in the first two to three years after menarche. Which patients should be evaluated? Generally the abrupt cessation of menses for four months after regular cycles or a history of oligomenorrhea and then four to six months of amenorrhea should be taken as a definite indication for an evaluation. Clearly many patients will present to the doctor after two, three, or eight months. Since the workup is simple and includes a physical exam, pregnancy test, and intramuscular progesterone, it should not be delayed until the patient fulfills arbitrary criteria.

On the other hand, if a sexually active patient is two weeks late for her period, intramuscular progesterone should not be used as a provocative test for pregnancy. A urine pregnancy test and physical exam are more appropriate. Progesterone will generally not induce a period in a patient with hypopituitarism secondary to a tumor or profound hypothalamic suppression seen with anorexia nervosa or massive weight gain, because the endometrium is not primed with estrogen. Most patients who do have withdrawal bleeding to progesterone are normal; however, disorders such as the Stein-Leventhal syndrome, ovarian tumors, thyroid disease, and diabetes should be excluded by physical examination and history. Provera, 10 mg orally for five days, may be substituted for intramuscular progesterone; however, if no withdrawal flow occurs, progesterone should be given before the physician proceeds to a more extensive evaluation. Galactorrhea should prompt an extensive neuroendocrine evaluation. Although an elevated LH (> 30 mIU/ml) and normal FSH may provide a clue to the diagnosis of Stein-Leventhal syndrome, serum gonadotropins are not necessary as part of the routine evaluation of secondary amenorrhea in a nonhirsute patient, at least at the present time. The evaluation of secondary amenorrhea is shown in Figure 6-8.

PREGNANCY

If the urine pregnancy test is negative in spite of a strong suspicion that the patient is pregnant (i.e., morning nausea, urinary frequency, breast soreness, and a slightly enlarged uterus), an ectopic pregnancy should be considered. A new serum test, the β-subunit HCG, detects very low levels of circulating human chorionic gonadotropin and is positive with ectopic pregnancy [12]. Laparoscopy is indicated in suspicious cases. (See also Chap. 10.)

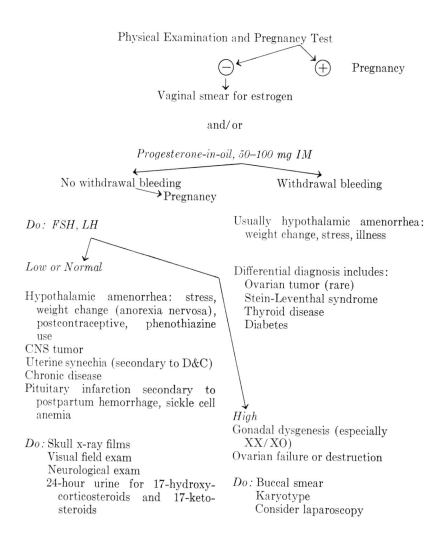

Physical Examination and Pregnancy Test

⊖ ← ⊕   Pregnancy

Vaginal smear for estrogen

and/or

Progesterone-in-oil, 50–100 mg IM

No withdrawal bleeding   Withdrawal bleeding
→ Pregnancy

Do: FSH, LH

Usually hypothalamic amenorrhea: weight change, stress, illness

Low or Normal

Hypothalamic amenorrhea: stress, weight change (anorexia nervosa), postcontraceptive, phenothiazine use
CNS tumor
Uterine synechia (secondary to D&C)
Chronic disease
Pituitary infarction secondary to postpartum hemorrhage, sickle cell anemia

Differential diagnosis includes:
Ovarian tumor (rare)
Stein-Leventhal syndrome
Thyroid disease
Diabetes

Do: Skull x-ray films
Visual field exam
Neurological exam
24-hour urine for 17-hydroxy-corticosteroids and 17-keto-steroids

High
Gonadal dysgenesis (especially XX/XO)
Ovarian failure or destruction

Do: Buccal smear
Karyotype
Consider laparoscopy

Fig. 6-8. Evaluation of secondary amenorrhea.

Withdrawal Flow to Intramuscular Progesterone

Hypothalamic amenorrhea

In most patients who have abundant, watery cervical mucus, a positive vaginal smear for estrogen, or a normal response to intramuscular progesterone, periods will return spontaneously without treatment. If the patient seems apprehensive, periods can be induced with Provera, 10 mg orally for five days every 6–12 weeks. Such cyclic therapy prevents endometrial hyperplasia secondary to prolonged estrogen stimulation and reassures the physician that the pituitary is producing FSH.

Birth control pills should not be used to cycle the patient artificially because these hormones continue the hypothalamic suppression.

In the well-estrogenized teenager, clomiphene can be used to initiate menses in the same dosages described on page 79. However, it is difficult to advocate the use of a drug that may result in hyperstimulation of the ovaries and that induces ovulation in a potentially sexually active teenager.

Stein-Leventhal syndrome

Definitions vary, but the Stein-Leventhal syndrome is usually defined as polycystic ovaries, oligomenorrhea or amenorrhea, and sterility. It is an infrequent cause of delayed menarche but a more common cause of secondary amenorrhea and later infertility. Some patients initially have regular periods and then later in adolescence develop secondary amenorrhea or oligomenorrhea, but the majority of patients have irregular periods starting with menarche. The majority are overweight; approximately 50 percent have hirsutism and a smaller percentage have definite virilization. Although in the past this diagnosis has usually been made in patients in their middle to late 20s, increasing awareness of this syndrome has resulted in earlier diagnosis.

The etiology of the syndrome is still in question. Although some investigators have demonstrated a partial block in estrogen synthesis with increased androstenedione production, most researchers have concluded that the hypothalamic-ovarian feedback mechanism is at fault [13]. Patients with so-called typical polycystic ovaries have elevated LH values (greater than 30 mIU/ml) and low or normal FSH values. Excess androgen and estrogen secretion presumably prevents the surge of LH at midcycle and instead induces constant release of LH throughout the cycle. Excess LH and perhaps insufficient FSH levels in turn induce constant excess ovarian estrogen and androgen production, leading to amenorrhea. It should be noted that peripheral conversion of androgen to estrogen also contributes to the elevated circulating estrogen levels. The ovaries enlarge with multiple cysts. The mechanism that induces this original imbalance and the possible role of the adrenal glands are as yet undefined. An "atypical" polycystic ovary syndrome has also been described with androgen excess, normal gonadotropins, and normal-size ovaries with thickened capsules. Proliferation of hyperplastic theca cells in the ovarian stroma (ovarian hyperthecosis) has been reported in a few adolescent patients with hirsutism and irregular periods [14].

Serum testosterone levels are often elevated in patients with polycystic ovaries, especially those with hirsutism or virilization. Urinary 17-ketosteroids may be normal or slightly to moderately elevated (15–25 mg/24 hours) and are usually only partially or not at all suppressible with dexamethasone [14, 15]. Diagnosis is usually confirmed by laparoscopy and ovarian biopsy.

Patients with normal-size ovaries (atypical polycystic ovary syndrome) but without evidence of hirsutism or virilization should be cycled with Provera, 10 mg every day for five days each month, to prevent endometrial hyperplasia. Patients with enlarged ovaries or androgen excess should be cycled with birth control pills to suppress the hypothalamic-ovarian axis. In most cases, patients should probably be continued on these pills until a pregnancy is desired.

Clomiphene citrate is an alternative form of therapy, which by its central action on the hypothalamus reverses the hormonal imbalance, perhaps by allowing LH to accumulate in the pituitary in adequate amounts to produce a midcycle surge. This drug should probably be reserved for use by gynecologists because of the risk of hyperstimulation of the polycystic ovaries. Clomiphene and/or wedge resection are used for patients desiring a pregnancy.

No withdrawal flow to intramuscular progesterone

LOW OR NORMAL FOLLICLE-STIMULATING AND LUTEINIZING HORMONE LEVELS

The conditions occurring with low or normal FSH and LH levels are CNS tumor (see p. 76), chronic disease (see p. 76), pituitary infarction, uterine synechia, and hypothalamic amenorrhea. The profound suppression of hypothalamic function in patients with anorexia nervosa and depression is responsible for the poor estrogenization; intramuscular progesterone or Provera will not induce a period in most of these patients. It is most important to exclude a CNS lesion and then direct therapy at the primary problem. Artificial cycling with Premarin/Provera or oral contraceptives is not indicated. In patients with profound weight loss, periods may not recommence for months, sometimes years, after the initial episode. Frisch [16] has shown that the mean weight for reestablishing menses is greater than the original mean weight at menarche. For example, the patient with a final height of 63 inches may weigh 91 pounds at menarche; if she loses weight and develops secondary amenorrhea, her periods may not resume until she achieves a weight of 102 pounds.

HIGH FOLLICLE-STIMULATING AND LUTEINIZING HORMONE LEVELS

Two conditions that occur with high FSH and LH levels are gonadal dysgenesis (see p. 72) and ovarian failure. Ovarian fibrosis and failure have been associated with cyclophosphamide (Cytoxan) therapy [17]. Patients with a history of prepubertal irradiation to the pelvis may occasionally develop secondary sexual characteristics and menses and later in adolescence present with secondary amenorrhea and ovarian failure. Patients with Addison's disease should be observed for the

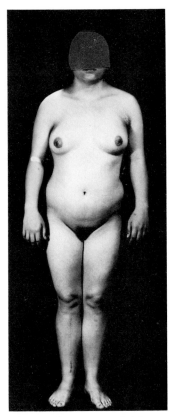

Fig. 6-9. Case 8: gonadal dysgenesis, XX/XO.

later development of autoimmune ovarian failure. In rare cases, ovarian destruction has followed a severe gonococcal infection.

Case 7. A. N., age 15, presented to the clinic with a history of fatigue. Further questioning revealed that her last menstrual period was two months previously. Her menarche was at age 12 and she had had regular cycles until the missed period. Although she initially denied the possibility of pregnancy, the Gravindex test was positive and her uterus was eight week size. After a therapeutic abortion, she decided to take oral contraceptive pills.

Case 8. B. D., age 17, presented to the clinic with a history of amenorrhea for six months. Breast and pubic hair development began at age 12. Menarche occurred at age 14, but she had only two to three periods each year. She denied sexual activity. On physical examination (Fig. 6–9) B. D. was a short young woman with several stigmata of Turner's syndrome (webbed neck, ptosis, low hairline, and short fourth metacarpals). Her height was 57¾ inches and her weight was 100 pounds. Breasts and pubic hair were stage V. Pelvic examination revealed a poorly estrogenized vagina with a small cervix and uterus; the vaginal smear showed no estrogen. The patient had no response to 100 mg intramuscular progesterone-in-oil. FSH was 197 mIU/ml and LH 150 mIU/ml; karyotype was XX/XO. She was placed on cyclic Premarin and Provera and had withdrawal flow each month.

SECONDARY AMENORRHEA AND HIRSUTISM AND/OR VIRILIZATION

The differential diagnosis of secondary amenorrhea and hirsutism and/or virilization includes the Stein-Leventhal syndrome, ovarian hyperthecosis, congenital (or adult-onset) adrenocortical hyperplasia, Cushing's syndrome, and ovarian and adrenal tumors. These entities are discussed in detail in the section on delayed menarche plus virilization in this chapter and in Chapter 13. The evaluation should include laboratory studies, such as a 24-hour urine test for 17-ketosteroids and 17-hydroxycorticosteroids; dexamethasone suppression test if the 17-ketosteroids are elevated; serum testosterone, 17-hydroxyprogesterone, FSH, and LH levels; and possibly laparoscopy. Referral to an endocrinologist is often necessary.

Case 9. D. V. presented to the clinic at age 19 with a history of amenorrhea for six months. Breast and pubic hair development began at age 13. She had her menarche at age 15 but never had more than two or three periods each year. Over the past few years she had noted progressive hirsutism. On physical examination D. V. was an overweight young woman with a height of 64 inches and a weight of 150 pounds. Blood pressure was 100/60; pulse was 74. She had moderate hirsutism with coarse, dark hair over her chin, chest, back, and extremities. Breast development was stage V. She had a normal pelvic exam without clitoromegaly. Urinary 17-ketosteroids were 24 and 32 mg/24 hours, suppressible with dexamethasone. Serum FSH, LH, and testosterone were within normal limits. An ACTH stimulation test was compatible with a partial 21-hydroxylase deficiency. On a maintenance dosage of dexamethasone, 0.5 mg at bedtime, the patient had good suppression of urinary 17-ketosteroids and regular menses.

OLIGOMENORRHEA

Teenagers with periods every two to three months often consult the physician for reassurance. Many teenage girls feel different from their friends who are having regular monthly cycles. Such periods may or may not be ovulatory. Premenstrual symptoms, dysmenorrhea, and a shift in the basal body temperature curve (see Chap. 1, p. 20) imply ovulation. Scanty, irregular periods without cramps are most likely anovulatory and often characterize the early teenage years.

A teenager of 16 or 17 years of age with oligomenorrhea deserves a careful general and pelvic examination to exclude systemic and gynecological problems (e.g., anorexia, hypothalamic amenorrhea, Stein-Leventhal syndrome), since irregular periods often precede secondary amenorrhea. Signs of hirsutism or androgen excess should prompt further laboratory tests. If the examination is normal, the patient deserves reassurance and a careful explanation of menstrual cycles. In general, the statement "You're normal; don't worry" is not sufficient. Patients should not be treated with oral contraceptives to produce "normal" cycles. Provera, 10 mg for the first five days of each month, can be used if the patient has a history of hypermenorrhea associated with the irregular periods.

Young women of 18 or 19 years of age, especially if concerned about future fertility, can be evaluated with basal body temperature charts and possibly an endometrial biopsy. Ovulatory cycles are indicated by a shift in the basal body temperature chart two weeks before the next menses. An endometrial biopsy done within 18 hours of the onset of menses provides confirmatory evidence of a shedding, secretory endometrium. If the cycles are ovulatory, the patient can be reassured. If the cycles are anovulatory, the patient may be cycled with Provera, 10 mg for five days each month. Clomiphene therapy (see p. 79) for three to four cycles can be used to induce ovulatory cycles with the hope that the patient will continue to cycle spontaneously after treatment. However, this medication runs the risk of an unwanted pregnancy and should for the most part be reserved for infertility patients under the care of a gynecologist.

If a young woman desires contraception and has a history of irregular anovulatory periods, the intrauterine device (IUD) or diaphragm should be suggested. However, if the pill seems to offer the only reliable mode of contraception, the patient should understand that she may have an increased risk of post-pill amenorrhea.

DYSFUNCTIONAL UTERINE BLEEDING: POLYMENORRHEA, HYPERMENORRHEA

One of the most common situations in the practice of adolescent medicine is the patient with irregular, profuse menstruation. Rarely, a teenager will with her first period show a decrease of 10 to 20 percentage points in her hematocrit. More usually a teenager who has had several years of regular cycles begins to have periods every two weeks or prolonged bleeding for 14–20 days. Young adolescents are prone to anovulatory periods with incomplete shedding of a proliferative endometrium; the older adolescent may develop anovulatory cycles with stress or illness. A recent study [18] of FSH/LH patterns in perimenarcheal dysfunctional bleeders suggests the prevalence of a maturation defect. The higher than normal levels of FSH in relation to LH may result in rapid follicular maturation and increased synthesis of estrogen, which may in turn prevent the midcycle surge of LH. Unopposed estrogen stimulation of the endometrium eventually results in irregular, painless, dysfunctional bleeding.

PATIENT EVALUATION

The evaluation of patients with irregular bleeding should include:

1. Physical examination, including speculum exam of the vagina and bimanual vaginal or rectal-abdominal palpation.
2. Complete blood count, including an estimate of platelets by smear.
3. Cervical culture for gonorrhea in sexually active adolescents.
4. Tine test.

A past history of painless irregular periods, especially if the interval between periods is less than 21 days, suggests anovulatory bleeding. Although a long list of diagnoses must be excluded before the assumption of dysfunctional bleeding is made, the history, physical exam, and response to therapy usually clarify the situation quickly. The differential diagnosis includes:

1. Missed abortion
2. Tubal pregnancy
3. Blood dyscrasias: decreased platelets, clotting disorders, iron deficiency
4. Endocrine: hypothyroidism or hyperthyroidism, adrenal disease, diabetes mellitus
5. Uterine: carcinoma (rare), fibroids, polyps
6. Vaginal: carcinoma, adenosis (secondary to maternal diethylstilbestrol)
7. Ovarian: Stein-Leventhal syndrome, tumors, pelvic inflammatory disease (PID), premature menopause
8. Systemic disease (e.g., tuberculosis)

If the uterus is soft or enlarged, pregnancy should be considered and a first morning urine should be screened for HCG. If the pregnancy test is negative or questionable and an adnexal mass is present, an ectopic pregnancy should be investigated. Patients with blood dyscrasias usually have other signs of bleeding (petechiae, ecchymoses, epistaxis); however, occasionally the teenager with chronic thrombocytopenic purpura or the cardiac patient on warfarin (Coumadin) may have profuse vaginal bleeding. It should be mentioned that iron deficiency may be a cause as well as a result of irregular bleeding.

The endocrine disorders of hypothyroidism and hyperthyroidism, adrenal disease, and diabetes are usually evident by history and physical exam; laboratory studies such as thyroxin (T_4), resin triiodothyronine (resin T_3), glucose, and urinary 17-ketosteroids and 17-hydroxycorticosteroids should be reserved for suggestive cases.

Carcinoma is a rare problem among teenagers; however, with the recent association of in utero exposure to diethylstilbestrol and the later development of vaginal and cervical adenocarcinoma in female offspring, it certainly behooves the physician to do a careful examination in patients with a positive maternal history (see Chap. 10). In addition, the fact that maternal histories are often inaccurate makes it important to examine all teenagers with irregular bleeding to exclude this rare problem. Ovarian tumors may also cause hypermenorrhea in the adolescent; most of these tumors are easily palpable on recto-abdominal examination (see Chap. 11).

Since irregular bleeding may be associated with gonorrhea or PID [19], an endocervical culture for gonococcus is indicated in all sexually active patients. Patients with cervical and adnexal tenderness should be evaluated with a sedimentation rate and treated for PID if indicated (see Chap. 9).

In the vast majority of cases, these diagnoses are readily excluded without an elaborate workup. The use of basal body temperature charts or an endometrial biopsy to confirm the diagnosis of anovulatory bleeding is usually unnecessary. Simple hormonal therapy will return most patients to regular cycles. Clinical suspicion or failure to respond to therapy should prompt further investigation.

TREATMENT

Although opinion clearly varies on the best mode of therapy, we have included the schedule that we have found helpful in our clinics.

For light to moderate vaginal bleeding of less than one month's duration or several months of very frequent periods (i.e., every one to three weeks), the treatment is Enovid-E (2.5 mg) twice a day for 10 days; or Ortho-Novum or Norinyl 2 mg twice a day for 10 days. If nausea or vomiting becomes a problem, tablets may be given once a day for 20 days. Bleeding should stop within a few days, and a normal withdrawal flow will follow two to four days after the last hormone tablet. The patient should then be cycled with Provera, 10 mg daily for the first five days of each month, for three to six months. If the patient has a history of many months of dysfunctional bleeding, she should probably be cycled on Enovid-E or Ortho-Novum 2 mg for two to three months, before initiating a six-month course of Provera.

For heavy vaginal bleeding (usually associated with anemia), an effective treatment is Ortho-Novum 2 mg or Enovid-E (2.5 mg) every 4 hours until bleeding slows or stops (usually four to eight tablets), then twice a day for the remainder of the package. A normal withdrawal flow follows two to four days after the last hormone tablet. The patient should then be cycled with Ortho-Novum 2 mg or Enovid-E for three to four months. If the regimen of hormone tablets every 4 hours fails to control bleeding within 36–48 hours, endometrial pathology should be excluded by dilation and curettage.

Patients with a long history of anovulatory cycles and dysfunctional bleeding have an increased risk of later infertility and endometrial carcinoma [20]. Therapy with Provera to induce a secretory endometrium and regular withdrawal flow may be needed on a long-term basis. Careful follow-up of these patients is essential.

REFERENCES

1. Engel, E., and Forbes, A.   Cytogenetic and clinical findings in 48 patients with congenitally defective or absent ovaries. *Medicine* (Baltimore) 44: 135, 1965.
2. McHardy-Young, S., et al.   Thyroid function in Turner's syndrome and allied conditions. *Lancet* 2:1161, 1970.
3. Ziel, H., and Finkle, W.   Increased risk of endometrial carcinoma among users of conjugated estrogens. *N. Engl. J. Med.* 293:1167, 1975.
4. Rothchild, E., and Owens, R.   Adolescent girls who lack functioning ovaries. *J. Am. Acad. Child Psychiatry* 11:88, 1972.
5. Frisch, R., and Nagel, L. S.   Prediction of adult height of girls from age of menarche and height at menarche. *J. Pediatr.* 85:838, 1974.
6. Jacobsen, A., et al.   Plasma gonadotropins during clomiphene-induced ovulatory cycles. *Am. J. Obstet. Gynecol.* 102:284, 1968.
7. Federman, D.   *Abnormal Sexual Development.* Philadelphia: Saunders, 1968.
8. Farber, M., and Marchant, D.   Congenital absence of the uterine cervix. *Am. J. Obstet. Gynecol.* 121:414, 1975.
9. Givens, J. R., et al.   Pseudohermaphroditism and deficient testicular 17-ketosteroid reductase. *N. Engl. J. Med.* 29:938, 1974.
10. Walsh, P. C., et al. Familial incomplete male pseudohermaphroditism, type 2. *N. Engl. J. Med.* 291:944, 1974.
11. Wilson, J. D., et al.   Familial incomplete male pseudohermaphroditism, type 1. *N. Engl. J. Med.* 290:1097, 1974.
12. Kosasa, T., et al.   Beta subunit HCG in the diagnosis of ectopic pregnancy. *Obstet. Gynecol.* 42:868, 1973.
13. DeVane, G. W., et al.   Circulating gonadotropins, estrogens, and androgens in polycystic ovary disease. *Am. J. Obstet. Gynecol.* 121: 496, 1975.
14. Wentz, A., et al.   Ovarian hyperthecosis in the adolescent patient. *J. Pediatr.* 88:488, 1976.
15. Easterling, E.   Serum testosterone levels in PCO. *Am. J. Obstet. Gynecol.* 120:385, 1974.
16. Frisch, R., and McArthur, J.   Menstrual cycles: Fatness as a determinant of minimal weight for height necessary for their maintenance or onset. *Science* 185:949, 1974.
17. Warne, G. L. Cyclophosphamide-induced ovarian failure. *N. Engl. J. Med.* 289:1159, 1973.
18. Ansel, S., and Jones, G.   Etiology and treatment of dysfunctional uterine bleeding. *Obstet. Gynecol.* 44:1, 1974.
19. Curran, J. W., et al.   Female gonorrhea: Its relation to abnormal uterine bleeding, urinary tract symptoms, and cervicitis. *Obstet. Gynecol.* 45:195, 1975.
20. Southam, A. L., and Richart, R. M.   The prognosis for adolescents with menstrual abnormalities. *Am. J. Obstet. Gynecol.* 94:637, 1966.

SUGGESTED READING

Aono, T., et al.   The diagnostic significance of LH-releasing hormone in patients with amenorrhea. *Am. J. Obstet. Gynecol.* 120:740, 1974.

Boyar, R., et al. Anorexia nervosa: Immaturity of LH secretory pattern. *N. Engl. J. Med.* 291:861, 1974.

Friedman, S. Clinical use of multiple serum FSH and LH measurements in patients with amenorrhea and infertility. *Obstet. Gynecol.* 41:809, 1973.

Gilson, M. D., and Knab, D. R. Primary amenorrhea: A simplified approach to diagnosis. *Am. J. Obstet. Gynecol.* 117:400, 1973.

Patton, W. C., et al. Pituitary gonadotropin response to synthetic LHRH in patients with typical and atypical polycystic ovary disease. *Am. J. Obstet. Gynecol.* 121:382, 1975.

Roth, J. C. FSH and LH response to LHRH in prepubertal and pubertal children, adult males and patients with hypogonadotropic and hyper-gonadotropic hypogonadism. *J. Clin. Endocrinol. Metab.* 35:926, 1972.

Serra, G. B. Enhancement of deficient pituitary response to LHRH in patients with primary amenorrhea. *Obstet. Gynecol.* 45:523, 1975.

Taymor, M., et al. LHRH as a diagnostic and research tool in gynecologic endocrinology. *Am. J. Obstet. Gynecol.* 120:721, 1974.

Wentz, A. C., et al. Gonadotropin responses following LHRH administration in normal subjects. *Obstet. Gynecol.* 45:239, 1975.

Wentz, A. C., et al. Diagnostic use of LHRH in primary amenorrhea. *Obstet. Gynecol.* 45:247, 1975.

Wentz, A. C., et al. Gonadotropin response to LHRH administration in secondary amenorrhea and galactorrhea syndromes. *Obstet. Gynecol.* 45:256, 1975.

Williams, R. *Textbook of Endocrinology* (5th ed.). Philadelphia: Saunders, 1974.

Yen, S. S. C., et al. Variation of pituitary responsiveness to synthetic LRF during different phases of the menstrual cycle. *J. Clin. Endocrinol. Metab.* 35:931, 1972.

7. Dysmenorrhea and Mittelschmerz

Dysmenorrhea is probably the most common gynecological complaint of adolescents. In typical histories the 14- or 15-year-old teenager, two to three years after her menarche, begins to develop crampy lower abdominal pain with each menstrual period. Usually the pains start within 1–4 hours of the onset of the period and last for about 24 hours. In some cases the pain may start one to two days before the period and continue for two to four days into the period. Nausea and vomiting and either diarrhea or constipation may accompany the cramps. Although the etiology of dysmenorrhea is unclear, the timing appears to coincide with the establishment of ovulatory cycles. Prostaglandins, released during menstrual breakdown of the endometrium, may play a role in stimulating contractility of the myometrium, which perhaps is sensitized by falling progesterone levels; this hypothesis is the rationale for utilizing antiprostaglandin drugs such as aspirin, indomethacin, and more recently the experimental drug flufenamic acid (Flunalgan)* [1]. Well over 95 percent of patients have functional dysmenorrhea, i.e., the examination is normal. A very small percentage of adolescents have organic pathology—chronic pelvic inflammatory disease, vaginal agenesis, rudimentary uterine horn, paramesonephric cysts, or endometriosis. In adolescents younger than age 17, endometriosis is uncommon and is usually associated with abnormal anatomy, such as cervical atresia or vaginal agenesis.

PATIENT EVALUATION

In assessing an adolescent with dysmenorrhea, the physician needs to know the patient's menstrual history, timing of the cramps, and premenstrual symptoms, as well as her response to the cramps. Key questions would be: Is she missing school? If so, how many days? Does she have nausea and vomiting? What medications has she used before? What is the nature of mother-daughter interaction? For the virginal girl of 13 or 14 who has mild cramps the first day of her period, a normal physical examination, including inspection of the genitalia to rule out an abnormality of the hymen, is reassuring. It is not necessary to do a vaginal exam. Treatment includes a careful explanation to the patient of the nature of the problem and a chance for her to ask questions regarding her anatomy. Mild analgesics, such as aspirin, acetaminophen (Tylenol), or Empirin, usually give adequate symptomatic relief.

* Rafa Laboratories Ltd., Jerusalem.

Patients with moderate or severe dysmenorrhea should have a pelvic exam. In the majority of adolescents who are carefully prepared, a vaginal exam is nontraumatic. In some patients a rectoabdominal exam is all that is possible, but even this will rule out adnexal tenderness and masses.

TREATMENT

If the exam is normal, treatment should be directed at symptomatic relief. Useful analgesics include aspirin, 300–600 mg every 4 hours; propoxyphene (Darvon), 65 mg every 6 hours; Empirin with 15–30 mg codeine, 1 tablet every 4 hours; or plain codeine, 30 mg every 4 hours. Although not as yet officially approved for dysmenorrhea, indomethacin (Indocin), 25 mg given three times daily with food, is an antiprostaglandin that has proved useful in several clinics. This medication is started at the first sign of the onset of the period and continued for two to three days or the usual duration of the cramps; it is not withheld until the patient has already experienced cramps.

Nausea and vomiting are best relieved by prochlorperazine (Compazine), 5–10 mg orally every 4 hours, started at the beginning of the period. Oral rather than rectal medications are tried first; if the patient vomits her pills, then a trial of chlorpromazine (Thorazine), 25 mg rectally every 6 hours, is warranted. Bed rest, a heating pad over the abdomen, and clear fluids are often useful adjuncts.

The adolescent should be seen every three to four months to evaluate the effectiveness of the medication. Such visits also facilitate doctor-patient rapport, which is essential in the treatment of this problem. Although some adolescents will use cramps as an excuse to stay out of school or to gain sympathy from the mother, patients should not be made to feel emotionally unstable because they complain of cramps. If the patient fails to respond to analgesics or indomethacin and continues to have severe pain and/or vomiting, she may be tried on a course of oral contraceptive pills, e.g., Norinyl 1/50, Ortho-Novum 1/50, or Ovral (see Chap. 14). A pelvic exam is necessary before this medication is instituted. Cramps should be relieved substantially, if not completely, with the anovulatory cycles and scantier flow. If severe cramps persist despite hormonal therapy, laparoscopy is indicated to rule out endometriosis or other organic causes before assuming that the etiology is emotional.

If dysmenorrhea is relieved, oral contraceptive pills are usually prescribed for three to six months and then discontinued. Often the patient will continue to have relief from cramps for several additional months. When cramps recur, analgesics and then oral contraceptives can be used again. Although a patient's symptoms sometimes seem to be secondary to a relative or functional cervical stenosis, cervical dilatation usually gives only temporary relief from dysmenorrhea and therefore should not be done on a routine basis.

PREMENSTRUAL SYMPTOMS

Premenstrual edema, bloating, and irritability may be complaints of the older teenager. In rare cases, the patient gains 10–15 pounds in the week before her period. The etiology is unclear, but the edema may result from sodium retention, which perhaps is related to high estrogen and progesterone levels.

Therapy is controversial and may be ineffective. Suggestions include:

1. Mild NaCl restriction.
2. Chlorothiazide (Diuril), 500 mg once or twice daily, the last week of the cycle (plus added K^+ as a glass of orange juice or banana daily).
3. For extreme irritability or nervousness, a mild tranquilizer may be used, e.g., diazepam (Valium), 5–10 mg three times daily, or chlordiazepoxide (Librium), 5 mg three times daily.

MITTELSCHMERZ

Mittelschmerz is the term applied to so-called ovulatory pain. The patient typically complains of dull, aching pain at midcycle in one lower quadrant, lasting from a few minutes to 6–8 hours. In rare instances the pain is described as severe and crampy and persists for two to three days. The etiology of this pain is unknown, but the spillage of fluid as the follicle cyst ruptures and expels the oocyte may irritate the peritoneum.

In most cases the diagnosis of mittelschmerz is evident from the recurrent nature of the mild discomfort. Documentation of the mid-cycle occurrence of the pain by menstrual charts is helpful. If the patient is being evaluated for the first episode or an exceptionally severe episode, other diagnoses must be excluded, including appendicitis, torsion or rupture of an ovarian cyst, and ectopic pregnancy. Laparoscopy is sometimes necessary to rule out serious pathology.

Therapy for mittelschmerz should aim foremost at a careful explanation to the teenager of the benign nature of the pain. A heating pad and analgesics may be indicated.

REFERENCE

1. Schwartz, A., et al. Primary dysmenorrhea. *Obstet. Gynecol.* 44:709, 1974.

SUGGESTED READING

Golub, L. Exercise and dysmenorrhea in young teenagers: A 3-year study. *Obstet. Gynecol.* 32:508, 1969.

Green, T. *Gynecology: Essentials of Clinical Practice* (3rd ed.). Boston: Little, Brown, 1977.

Huffman, J. *The Gynecology of Childhood and Adolescence*. Philadelphia: Saunders, 1969.

Ogden, J., et al.   Treatment of dysmenorrhea. *Am. J. Obstet. Gynecol.* 106: 838, 1970.

8. Vulvovaginitis in the Adolescent

In the adolescent, vaginitis represents a common gynecological problem despite the development of a more resistant, estrogenized vaginal epithelium, pubic hair, and labial fat pads. The striking difference between prepubertal and adolescent vaginitis is the shift in etiology. Vulvovaginitis in the prepubertal child is usually nonspecific—a mixed flora of *Escherichia coli*, *Streptococcus*, *Pseudomonas*, and *Proteus*—and results from poor perineal hygiene; whereas vaginitis in the adolescent usually has a specific etiology, often related to sexual contact—e.g., gonorrhea, *Trichomonas*, *Candida*, *Hemophilus vaginalis*, herpes. In addition to these true infections, the most common cause of discharge in the pubescent girl is probably physiological leukorrhea, a normal desquamation of epithelial cells secondary to estrogen effect.

PATIENT EVALUATION

The diagnosis of a vaginal discharge should include a history of symptoms (pruritus, odor, quantity), other illnesses (e.g., diabetes), and recent medications (e.g., broad spectrum antibiotics, birth control pills). The patient should be questioned about recent sexual relations, since treatment failure in the adolescent girl is often secondary to reinfection from an untreated contact. It should be remembered that several infections may coexist; for example, a patient may be treated adequately for *Trichomonas* and yet have a persistent malodorous discharge secondary to *H. vaginalis*. Another patient may have gonorrhea, *Trichomonas*, and scabies. Not infrequently in the evaluation of a vaginitis, the patient is found to be in need of birth control as well. The presence of *Trichomonas*, condyloma, lice, or herpes does not, however, necessarily imply sexual relations, since close family contact can spread these infections. A history of broad spectrum antibiotic therapy or uncontrolled diabetes is frequently a clue to the diagnosis of a monilial vaginitis.

The evaluation of a vaginal discharge in the adolescent usually requires a pelvic examination, saline and potassium hydroxide (KOH) preparations (described in Chapter 1), and sometimes cultures. The appearance of the vulva may be helpful in the differential diagnosis. Patients with acute monilial vulvovaginitis characteristically have a red, edematous vulva; patients with subacute or chronic moniliasis often have fissures, excoriation, and secondary bacterial infections. Small vesicles or ulcers associated with inguinal adenopathy are typical of herpetic vulvitis. The wet preparations usually provide the key to diagnosis. The saline preparation shows dancing, flagellated organisms in *Trichomonas* infections, epithelial cells without much evidence of inflammation in physiological leukorrhea, and so-called clue cells (epithelial cells coated with refractile bacteria) in an *H. vaginalis* infection. The KOH preparation is used to demonstrate the budding hyphae of *Candida*. The endocervix should be cultured for gonorrhea in all sexually active teenagers. A culture for *Candida* on Nickerson's media is helpful if the discharge is itchy and cheesy and yet no hyphae are seen on the KOH preparation.

To facilitate diagnosis and treatment, the various types of vaginitis are presented in this chapter. In most situations, the following non-specific therapy should also be included:

1. Warm baths twice a day (baking soda may be added if the vulva is irritated). Only bland soaps should be used.
2. Careful drying after the bath and application of baby powder to the vulva.
3. Frequent changes of white cotton underpants to absorb the discharge.
4. Good perineal hygiene (including wiping from front to back after bowel movements).
5. Avoidance of chemical douches and bubble bath. If a patient insists on douching, suggest plain warm water or ¼ cup white vinegar per quart of warm water.

TYPES OF VAGINITIS

TRICHOMONAL VAGINITIS

AGENT: *Trichomonas*, a small, flagellated parasite.

SYMPTOMS: Frothy, malodorous, yellow discharge that may cause itching and burning in the vulvar area. May be asymptomatic and found on routine Papanicolaou smear or wet preparation.

SOURCE: Usually venereal. Males are usually asymptomatic but may reinfect the female after she is treated.

DIAGNOSIS: On wet preparation of the discharge, flagellated organisms are visible dancing under the microscope. The cervix and vagina may show small punctate hemorrhagic spots.

TREATMENT: Metronidazole (Flagyl), 2 gm all in one dose [1]; *or* 250 mg orally three times daily for 7 days; *or* 500 mg orally twice a day for five days. Treat partner at the same time. Instruct patient to avoid alcohol (Flagyl and alcohol may lead to vomiting) and intercourse during the course of medication.

Clotrimazole (Gyne-Lotrimin), 100 mg vaginal tablets, 1 at bedtime for seven nights, appears to offer effective alternative treatment.

FOR RECURRENT INFECTIONS: Repeat course of oral Flagyl or vaginal Gyne-Lotrimin and make sure partner(s) is/are treated.

PREGNANCY: Local measures such as douching, Aci-Jel, AVC cream, or Gyne-Lotrimin (second and third trimesters) should be tried first. The partner should be treated with Flagyl orally (as previously described). Although no birth defects have been associated with Flagyl, it is contraindicated in the first trimester of pregnancy and should be used in the second and third trimesters only in patients in whom the local measures suggested previously are inadequate.

MONILIAL VAGINITIS

AGENT: *Candida albicans.*

SYMPTOMS: Thick, cheesy, extremely pruritic discharge. Vulva may be red and edematous.

SOURCE: Occasionally venereal. *Candida* may be present asymptomatically and then become the predominant organism during pregnancy, hormonal therapy, or after a course of broad spectrum antibiotics such as ampicillin or tetracycline. Diabetics, especially those with poor control, are prone to recurrent infections.

DIAGNOSIS: On KOH preparation, budding hyphae are present. In questionable cases, the diagnosis may be confirmed with the use of Nickerson's medium. In addition, growth of *Candida* also frequently occurs on Transgrow* and Thayer-Martin media, which are used for gonococcal cultures.

TREATMENT: Sitz baths with baking soda but no soap. Miconazole (Monistat) vaginal cream, 1 applicatorful at bedtime for 14 nights; *or* clotrimazole (Gyne-Lotrimin), 100-mg vaginal tablets, 1 at bedtime for seven nights.

  Alternates: Nystatin (Mycostatin) vaginal suppositories, 1 twice daily for 14 days; *or* Sporostacin vaginal cream, 1 applicatorful twice daily for 14 days; *or* candicidin (Candeptin, Vanobid) vaginal tablets, 1 twice daily for 14 days; *or* gentian violet jellies, creams, or tampons (Gentia-Jel, Gentersel cream, Genapax), 1 applicatorful or 1 tampon at bedtime for 12–24 nights (stains underwear).

  Although more expensive, miconazole cream has resulted in higher cure rates than traditionally prescribed nystatin, especially for pregnant patients and those taking oral contraceptive pills [2]. In patients with severe vulvitis, the addition of hydrocortisone cream 1% plus nystatin cream applied three times daily to the vulvar area for three to seven days gives marked symptomatic relief. These may be prescribed separately or in combination (Nystaform, Mycolog).

FOR RECURRENT INFECTIONS: Treat with one of the above for 30 days through a menstrual period or apply gentian violet 1% to cervix

* Scott Laboratories, Fiskeville, R.I. 02823.

and vagina every two to three days for three or four treatments. Then have the patient use a vinegar douche (¼ cup white vinegar per quart of water) *or* Aci-Jel vaginal jelly, 1 applicatorful at the end of each period for two to three days, at the first sign of itching, and whenever broad spectrum antibiotics are prescribed.

Nystatin, 500,000 units orally twice daily for 10 days, reduces colonic colonization with *Candida* and may prevent reinfections. In recurrent monilial infections, urinalysis and perhaps a two-hour postprandial glucose or glucose tolerance test should be done to rule out diabetes mellitus.

Nonspecific Vaginitis

AGENT: Although difficult to prove, most bacterial nonspecific vaginitis is probably secondary to *H. vaginalis* (a pleomorphic gram-negative coccobacillus).

SYMPTOMS: An irritating gray or clear discharge and typical "fishy" smell are associated with *H. vaginalis* infection.

SOURCE: Occasional venereal origin.

DIAGNOSIS: On wet preparation, large epithelial cells coated with small refractile bacteria (so-called clue cells) are visible. Polymorphonuclear cells are often present. Although cultures are usually unnecessary, *H. vaginalis* can be isolated by streaking the discharge on chocolate agar and incubating the plate under increased carbon dioxide tension.

TREATMENT: Sultrin Triple Sulfa cream, 1 applicatorful twice daily, or vaginal tablets, 1 twice daily for seven to ten days; *or* AVC cream, 1 applicatorful twice daily for two weeks. If local treatment for *H. vaginalis* fails, systemic therapy should be given: ampicillin, 500 mg four times daily, or tetracycline, 500 mg four times daily for ten days. The patient may benefit from the use of Aci-Jel vaginally while on systemic antibiotics to prevent a secondary monilial vaginitis.

Gonorrhea

AGENT: Neisseria gonorrhoeae.

SYMPTOMS: Often asymptomatic. In symptomatic patients, a purulent discharge from the cervical os.

SOURCE: Sexual contact.

DIAGNOSIS: Culture on Thayer-Martin or Transgrow media. Gram's stain of the discharge may reveal gram-negative intracellular diplococci (suggestive but not conclusive evidence in women because of the possible presence of saprophytic *Neisseria*).

TREATMENT: See Chapter 9.

Leukorrhea

AGENT: A normal estrogen effect.

SYMPTOMS: A whitish discharge that usually starts before the menarche and may continue for several years.

DIAGNOSIS: The wet preparation reveals epithelial cells without evidence of inflammation.

TREATMENT: Good perineal hygiene, including frequent washing with mild soap and warm water; cotton underpants (frequent changes); reassurance.

Nonspecific Vulvitis

AGENT: A nonspecific vulvar irritation may be caused by hot weather, nylon underpants, obesity, poor hygiene, or sand from sunbathing.

SYMPTOMS: Pruritus, pain, dysuria.

DIAGNOSIS: By history, and exclusion of a specific vaginitis.

TREATMENT: Hydrocortisone cream 1% applied three times daily to the vulva; white cotton underpants; avoidance of precipitating factors.

Condyloma Acuminatum

AGENT: Probably a virus.

SYMPTOMS: Wartlike growths on vulva and vagina; occasional dyspareunia.

SOURCE: Close physical contact. Lesions are often associated with a specific vaginitis.

DIAGNOSIS: Inspection. A serum Venereal Disease Research Laboratory test should be done to rule out syphilis.

TREATMENT: Clearing the vaginitis will often lead to the spontaneous disappearance of these warts. If the warts are treated as described below without clearing the vaginitis, they will tend to recur.

Apply podophyllin resin (25%) in tincture of benzoin to the small lesions, carefully avoiding the normal skin. If the lesions are numerous, a few can be treated each week. The patient is instructed to take a bath and wash her perineum well two hours after the podophyllin therapy. If she experiences a local burning sensation, petroleum jelly or lidocaine (Xylocaine) jelly 2% may give symptomatic relief. Additional treatment is given every one to two weeks as needed. Lesions should not be treated with podophyllin during pregnancy because of systemic absorption. If the lesions are large (greater than 1 cm), excision, fulguration, or cryocautery is usually indicated.

The patient should understand that the warts may recur and need retreatment.

HERPES VULVITIS

AGENT: Herpes simplex, type 2.

SYMPTOMS: Local burning and irritation, dysuria. Vesicles appear on the labia, vagina, and/or cervix and then rupture within one to three days, producing painful small ulcers that may be super-infected with gram-negative organisms or *Candida*. Inguinal adenopathy and fever may be present.

SOURCE: Venereal (currently the second most common venereal disease in the United States). Thirty percent of cases are new infections; 70 percent are recurrences.

DIAGNOSIS: Inspection. A scraping of the base of the lesion stained with Wright's stain will reveal multinucleate giant cells and inclusions. Viral cultures are usually not necessary or possible in practice.

TREATMENT: Lesions disappear spontaneously within ten days to four weeks, although they may recur.

SYMPTOMATIC TREATMENT: Warm baths; Betadine aqueous solution 1%, applied three times daily with cotton balls or douche [3], and/or Xylocaine jelly 2% applied four times daily.

   Although photodynamic therapy with proflavine or neutral red dye and subsequent exposure to light appears to shorten the duration of symptoms and prevent recurrences, concern has been expressed that this treatment might contribute to the oncogenic potential of the herpes virus and therefore is not recommended. Patients with herpetic infections have an increased risk of later developing cervical cancer. Pregnant patients who have active herpes infections at term should be delivered by cesarean section because of the risk of disseminated herpes in the newborn.

PEDICULOSIS PUBIS (CRABS)

AGENT: *Phthirius pubis* (crab lice).

SYMPTOMS: Pruritus.

SOURCE: Close physical contact; infested blankets and clothing.

DIAGNOSIS: On inspection, minute, firmly attached flakes (1–2 mm) are visible on the pubic hair. Under the low-power microscope, the flakes are adult lice or nits.

TREATMENT: 1% gamma benzene hexachloride (Kwell) shampoo; re-peat in 24 hours. Clothing and blankets should be laundered or dry cleaned.

PINWORMS

AGENT: *Enterobius vermicularis* (pinworm).

SYMPTOMS: Pruritus, mostly around the anus.

SOURCE: Oral-anal spread, more common in young children.

DIAGNOSIS: A piece of Scotch tape is blotted around the anus as soon as the patient awakes in the morning. The tape is affixed to a glass slide and is examined for the presence of typical ova. Rarely, an adult pinworm may be seen in the vagina.

TREATMENT: See page 39.

VAGINITIS SECONDARY TO A FOREIGN BODY

AGENT: In adolescents, usually a retained tampon.

SYMPTOMS: Foul-smelling, often bloody discharge.

DIAGNOSIS: Examination.

TREATMENT: Removal of the foreign body and irrigation of the vagina with warm water.

REFERENCES

1. Dykers, J. Single dose metronidazole for *Trichomonas:* Patient and consort. *N. Engl. J. Med.* 293:23, 1975.
2. Davis, J., et al. Comparative evaluation of Monistat and Mycostatin in the treatment of vulvovaginal candidiasis. *Obstet. Gynecol.* 44:403, 1974.
3. Friedrich, E., and Masukawa, T. Effect of povidone-iodine on herpes genitalis. *Obstet. Gynecol.* 45:337, 1975.

SUGGESTED READING

Barchet, S. A new look at vaginal discharges. *Obstet. Gynecol.* 40:615, 1972.
Green, T. *Gynecology: Essentials of Clinical Practice* (3rd ed.). Boston: Little, Brown, 1977.
Altchek, A. Adolescent vulvovaginitis. *Pediatr. Clin. North Am.* 19(3):735, 1972.

9. Venereal Disease

GONOCOCCAL INFECTIONS

School lectures, popular magazines, and scientific journals currently point to the epidemic increase in reported cases of gonococcal infections. The increase is probably the result of many factors, including earlier sexual relations among teenagers, decreased use of the condom, increased health facilities for teenagers allowing better treatment and reporting, and the recognition of asymptomatic infections in males and females. Last year the United States had approximately one million reported cases and perhaps two million unreported cases of gonorrhea. The incidence of all cases of gonorrhea was highest among women 20–24 years old, with women in the 15- to 19-year-old age group second. However, the incidence of disseminated infection including pelvic inflammatory disease and arthritis was greatest among 15- to 19-year-old women.

Isolating *Neisseria gonorrhoeae*, a fastidious gram-negative diplococcus, requires special techniques. Culture swabs should always be planted directly on the appropriate medium. Thayer-Martin plates must be immediately transported to a suitable laboratory and incubated under increased carbon dioxide tension. Two new alternatives, Transgrow* and Modified Thayer Martin-Jembec†, offer selective media that have the advantage of easy transportation and mailing. Transgrow bottles should be held upright when the swab is streaked over the agar; isolation of the gonococcus is slightly improved if the medium is incubated at 37° C for 12–18 hours before mailing.

In most cases gonorrhea is a local infection. Screening cervical cultures indicates that the asymptomatic rate of gonorrhea ranges from 0.2 to 13 percent in adult women, depending on the setting. Private practices show significantly lower rates than large outpatient hospital clinics. However, the low rate of 0.2 percent should not reassure the physician who is seeing sexually active teenagers. "Nice girls don't get gonorrhea" is an unfortunate myth. No large study has documented rates of infection among teenage girls except in delinquent homes where the asymptomatic rate may range from 10 to 12 percent [1, 2].

Probably 80–90 percent of all gonococcal infections in women and 10–40 percent of infections in males are asymptomatic. Although culturing the endocervix, rectum, and pharynx may seem optimal, a single endocervical culture will pick up approximately 70–85 percent of cases of gonorrhea. On the basis of cost-benefit analysis, rectal and pharyngeal cultures should probably be done on a selective basis only [3].

* Scott Laboratories, Fiskeville, R.I. 02823.
† Gibco, Madison, Wisc. 53713.

CERVICITIS

The presenting complaints of patients with gonococcal cervicitis include a vaginal discharge, dysuria, urinary frequency, and dyspareunia. On examination, the cervix is typically tender to palpation; Gram's stain of the purulent discharge may reveal many polymorphonuclear cells with gram-negative intracellular diplococci. Since saprophytic *Neisseria* may be present in the vagina, the diagnosis of gonorrhea must be confirmed by culture. However, treatment can be initiated on the basis of symptoms and a positive smear.

PROCTITIS

An occasional patient with symptomatic low-grade proctitis will have positive gonorrhea culture and respond to appropriate therapy.

Treatment of asymptomatic infections, contacts,
cervicitis, and proctitis

The preferred treatment is aqueous procaine penicillin G,* 4.8 million units intramuscularly, divided into two doses and injected into two different sites at one visit, and probenecid, 1 gm given orally just before the injections. Alternatives to this treatment are:

1. Ampicillin, 3.5 gm orally (all in one dose in the presence of a nurse) and probenecid, 1 gm given simultaneously.
2. Tetracycline, 1.5 gm stat. and then 500 mg four times a day for four days (total dosage 9.5 gm).
3. Spectinomycin, 2 gm intramuscularly.
4. Erythromycin, 1.5 gm stat. and then 500 mg four times a day for four days.

Effective therapy for pregnant patients includes procaine penicillin, ampicillin, and probably erythromycin. Tetracycline should not be used to treat pregnant patients. The safety of spectinomycin for the fetus has not yet been established.

Patients are instructed to abstain from sexual relations for seven days and to return for a repeat cervical and rectal (pharyngeal) culture 7–14 days after treatment. Most positive cultures on follow-up are probably the result of reinfection. True treatment failures should be given spectinomycin, 2 gm intramuscularly.

A serology for syphilis should be performed prior to therapy. Procaine penicillin G will adequately treat incubating syphilis (negative serology); however, the other treatment regimens may not be suffi-

---

* Although penicillin is the treatment of choice, procaine has been reported to precipitate behavioral and neurological reactions—auditory and visual disturbances, dizziness, palpitation, twitching, seizures, and fear of death—in 0.9 percent of patients in one venereal disease clinic [4].

cient and thus a follow-up serum test should be performed three months after alternative treatment.

Every patient should be interviewed for contacts for the pertinent interval of duration of symptoms plus 14 days (30 days if possible). Regardless of symptoms, all contacts should be cultured and treated at the same visit.

PHARYNGITIS

The incidence of symptomatic and asymptomatic pharyngitis among teenagers is unknown. Gonococcal pharyngitis is related to the practice of fellatio. Although some reports suggest that the symptomatic patient has a red, edematous vulva with vesiculopustular lesions on the soft palate and tonsillar pillars, a characteristic clinical picture probably does not exist [5]. Diagnosis is by culture on appropriate media. Treatment is with procaine penicillin G and probenecid or tetracycline as described in the previous section. Ampicillin and spectinomycin are not adequate therapy.

VULVOVAGINITIS

Gonococcal infection in the prepubertal girl is usually a purulent vulvovaginitis rather than a cervicitis. Sexual or close family contacts are the source of the gonorrhea. Child abuse should be considered.

The preferred treatment is procaine penicillin G, 100,000 units/kg intramuscularly, and, if the patient is more than 2 years old, probenecid, 25 mg/kg orally just before the injection. Alternative treatment is erythromycin, 40 mg/kg/day divided into four doses for seven days (for patients under the age of 8); tetracycline 25 mg/kg stat. and then 40–60 mg/kg/day divided into four doses for seven days (for patients older than age 8).

A follow-up culture should be done seven days after therapy. The source of the infection should be identified and treated. A serology for syphilis should be done prior to therapy.

PELVIC INFLAMMATORY DISEASE (PID)

The menstrual period is often a precipitating factor in the dissemination of gonococcal disease. During the menses gonococci may ascend to the endometrium and fallopian tubes, resulting in the classic picture of acute salpingitis—acute lower abdominal pain, vaginal discharge, fever, and chills. Not infrequently less specific symptoms may herald the onset of salpingitis, e.g., menstrual irregularities, vomiting, diarrhea or constipation, dysuria, and urinary frequency. Physical findings on pelvic examination include pain on motion of the cervix and bilateral adnexal tenderness, sometimes with signs of peritoneal irritation or a mass. Gram's stain of the purulent cervical discharge may reveal gram-negative intracellular diplococci (with the same limitations as noted on p. 114). The white blood cell count may be normal or elevated; the sedimentation rate is greater than 15 mm/hour in 75–85 percent of patients. Gonorrhea is cultured from the endocervix in 40–60 percent of cases of acute salpingitis; *Mycoplasma*, coliforms, enterococci, streptococci, *Staphylococcus aureas,* and a variety of anaerobic organisms (*Bacteroides fragilis, Peptostreptococcus,* and *Peptococcus*) are probably responsible for most cases of nongonococcal PID [6, 7, 8].

The differential diagnosis is sometimes difficult. Laparoscopic studies of patients with a presumptive diagnosis of acute salpingitis have concluded that the clinical diagnosis is confirmed by visual inspection in only 60–70 percent of cases. An additional 5 percent of patients with negative exams by laparoscopy do, however, have gonorrhea by cervical culture. Jacobson found that 12 percent of patients with "clinical PID" had a different diagnosis: acute appendicitis, ectopic pregnancy, ruptured corpus luteum, ovarian abscess, or endometriosis [9, 10]. Acute appendicitis, often considered in the differential diagnosis, is usually associated with unilateral signs and symptoms and a normal sedimentation rate. If the diagnosis is in doubt, laparoscopy or laparotomy, depending on the skill of the surgeon, is indicated.

Inpatient therapy for acute pelvic inflammatory disease

The majority of patients with acute salpingitis should be admitted to the hospital. Certainly all cases with a questionable diagnosis, suspected pelvic abscess, peritoneal signs, or complications (including pregnancy) deserve admission. Cultures for gonorrhea and, if feasible, *Mycoplasma* should be done prior to antibiotic therapy. Preferred treatment includes bedrest in a semi-Fowler's position, and ampicillin, 1 gm intravenously every 4 hours until the patient has been afebrile for 48 hours. Alternative therapy is tetracycline, 500 mg every 6 hours intravenously or orally (preferably orally if tolerated). Ambulation is then permitted, and intravenous ampicillin therapy is continued for an additional 24 hours. If the temperature remains normal, oral ampicillin, 500 mg four times a day, can be started, and the patient may be discharged 48 hours later. Oral antibiotics should be continued and the patient seen weekly until the sedimentation rate has returned to normal.

Some patients fail to respond within 36–48 hours to intravenous ampicillin. This problem may result from a *Mycoplasma* or mixed anaerobic and aerobic bacterial peritoneal infection. In these instances tetracycline, 500 mg every 6 hours intravenously or orally, *or* chloramphenicol, 50–100 mg/kg/day (up to 2 gm/day) intravenously, should be added. The best antibiotic for this purpose is still a matter of controversy.

During the course of the infection the fallopian tubes may become occluded, producing a hydrosalpinx or pyosalpinx. Such masses discovered on initial pelvic exam should be followed carefully in the hospital. Surgery is rarely indicated unless the patient fails to improve clinically or the danger of spontaneous rupture becomes significant.

Outpatient therapy of acute pelvic inflammatory disease

The reliable patient who has mild symptoms, a temperature less than 100.5° F, and no peritoneal signs on physical examination may be treated as an outpatient. Treatment includes bed rest for 48 hours and tetracycline, 1.5 gm stat. and then 500 mg four times a day for 14 days or until the sedimentation rate is normal, *or* if the smear is positive, procaine penicillin G, 4.8 million units intramuscularly, and probenecid, 1 gm given orally just before the injections, followed by ampicillin, 500 mg four times daily for 14 days or until the sedimentation rate is normal.

Follow-up of acute pelvic inflammatory disease

Patients are instructed to avoid intercourse for three to four weeks. In gonorrhea-positive patients, repeat cervical and rectal cultures should be obtained one week after discontinuing antibiotics. Contacts should be treated to prevent reinfection.

Infertility, ectopic pregnancies, and chronic abdominal pain are the principal sequelae of acute PID. Tubal occlusion is more common in nongonococcal infections. In a recent study of laparoscopically-proved PID, tubal occlusion was verified after one infection in 12.8 percent of patients, after two infections in 35.5 percent, and after three or more infections in 75 percent [11].

Subacute and chronic pelvic inflammatory disease

PID may also be a subacute or chronic process; the patient usually complains of chronic bilateral or unilateral lower abdominal pain. The physical examination may reveal mild adnexal tenderness or a mass (hydrosalpinx). The sedimentation rate may be normal or slightly elevated. Routine cervical cultures are often negative for pathogenic organisms; *Mycoplasma* or a mixed flora of gram-negative and positive bacteria may be responsible for the "smoldering" salpingitis. Thus, if feasible, a *Mycoplasma* culture from patient (and partner) should be obtained prior to therapy.

Laparoscopy is often necessary to establish the diagnosis and to evaluate the extent of the disease. Subacute PID is characterized by serosal inflammation without masses; in chronic PID there are adhesions, masses, and thickenings in the base of the broad ligaments.

Therapy must be individualized. In patients with subacute PID, tetracycline, 500 mg four times a day, should be given for 14 days or until the sedimentation rate is normal (if initially elevated). Alternative treatment (if *Mycoplasma* culture is negative) is ampicillin, 500 mg four times a day for 14 days. In patients with chronic PID and frequent exacerbations, a six-month course of suppressive antibiotics should be tried, e.g., tetracycline 250 mg four times daily. Patients with chronic PID and relatively few flare-ups should be treated for each acute episode with tetracycline or ampicillin, 500 mg four times daily for 14 days.

Conservative surgery (presacral neurectomy, lysis of adhesions) may be necessary in patients with recurrent severe pain that is unresponsive to antibiotic therapy. In rare instances, hysterectomy may be the only definitive treatment.

ARTHRITIS

The diagnosis of gonococcal arthritis depends largely on suspicion because the source of the gonococcus in adolescent girls is usually an asymptomatic or low-grade cervicitis. Two forms of gonococcal arthritis have been described by Holmes and other authors [12, 13]. The "early" form classically begins at the onset of or just following a menstrual period and is characterized by migratory polyarthralgias, tenosynovitis, fever, chills, and skin lesions (pinpoint erythematous papules that may progress to purpuric vesiculopustular lesions). Blood cultures are usually positive if taken within two days of the onset of symptoms. Joint fluid, usually scanty, is negative for the gonococcus.

The "late" form of gonococcal arthritis is characterized by a monoarticular effusion, most often involving the knee, with a positive synovial fluid culture in 20–50 percent of cases. Blood cultures are negative and systemic symptoms are usually minimal.

Treatment consists of aqueous penicillin G, 2.5 million units intravenously every 6 hours, for three days or until significant clinical improvement occurs. A longer course of therapy may not be necessary but may be provided with ampicillin, 500 mg orally four times a day, for a total of seven days of antibiotic therapy. Alternative therapy is ampicillin, 3.5 gm given orally, plus probenecid, 1 gm orally, followed by ampicillin, 500 mg orally four times a day for seven days; *or* tetracycline, 1.5 gm stat., then 500 mg four times daily for seven days; *or* erythromycin, 500 mg intravenously every 6 hours for at least three days.

Hospitalization is indicated for unreliable patients and those with purulent joint effusions or uncertain diagnosis. Immobilization of the joint is probably helpful. Open drainage of joints other than the hip is usually unnecessary [14, 15].

MISCELLANEOUS

Gonococcal endocarditis and meningitis have been reported. Meningitis should be treated with penicillin, 10 million units/day intravenously for at least 10 days; endocarditis with penicillin, 10–20 million units/ day intravenously for four weeks.

SYPHILIS

The incidence of syphilis has also increased in the past decade for reasons similar to those discussed in the section on gonorrhea. Screening sexually active teenagers once a year with a serum Venereal Disease Research Laboratory test (VDRL) may pick up unsuspected cases. Current laws require a Hinton test, VDRL, or similar reagin test prior to marriage and with each pregnancy. Any patient with a suspicious oral or genital lesion or an unexplained generalized skin rash should have a serological test for syphilis.

A darkfield examination should be done by an experienced physician on the exudate from the lesion. The finding of *Treponema pallidum* under the microscope is diagnostic of syphilis; a positive VDRL or Hinton test is presumptive evidence of past or present infection with syphilis. False positive reagin tests occur in 1 out of 3,000 to 5,000 healthy patients. Infections such as mononucleosis, hepatitis, malaria, vaccinia, and collagen diseases may result in a false positive VDRL. If the clinical evidence does not favor the diagnosis, a treponemal antibody test (FTA-ABS) is indicated. The FTA-ABS is positive in most stages of syphilis, and only a few false positive results have been reported in patients with elevated globulins [16].

STAGES OF SYPHILIS

The stages of syphilis are as follows:

1. Primary syphilis: Ten to ninety days (average three weeks) after oral or genital exposure to an infected partner, the young woman may develop a hard, painless chancre on her vulva, vagina, cervix, or more rarely the mouth. Not infrequently the lesions are asymptomatic and may be missed; inguinal adenopathy may be present. The serological test for syphilis becomes positive five to six weeks after exposure; thus, a negative test at the time a lesion is noted does not rule out the diagnosis. A darkfield examination of the clear fluid expressed from the chancre should be done by an experienced physician and is diagnostic if positive. If negative, the darkfield examination should be repeated for three consecutive days. Even without therapy, the lesion(s) will heal spontaneously.

2. Secondary syphilis: If the chancre is untreated, the patient may experience, six weeks to several months later, the symptoms of secondary syphilis, including a generalized maculopapular or papulosquamous rash (often present on the palms and soles), fever, malaise, alopecia, weight loss, lymphadenopathy, condylomata lata, or mucous membrane lesions. The serum VDRL at this time is always positive; a spinal fluid VDRL is also positive in about 25 percent of such cases.

3. Latent syphilis: By definition, this is the stage of syphilis in which the patient has no symptoms and the spirochete is "hidden." However, the patient may be infectious and may later develop symptoms of tertiary syphilis. This stage is divided into early latent (less than 2 years of symptoms) and late latent (more than 2 years of symptoms).

4. Late syphilis: Except for gummas which are probably a hypersensitivity phenomenon, the late manifestations of syphilis (neurological and cardiovascular problems) are the result of a vasculitis. This diagnosis is usually made in patients well beyond the adolescent age group, although very rarely neurosyphilis or cardiovascular lesions can develop in adolescents as a sequela of untreated congenital syphilis.

TREATMENT WITH PENICILLIN

Primary or secondary syphilis or contact history

Benzathine penicillin G, 2.4 million units intramuscularly (1.2 million units in each buttock), should be given twice at one-week intervals; *or* aqueous procaine penicillin G, 600,000 units intramuscularly for 10 days, can be given (current recommendations of the Massachusetts Department of Health).

Latent syphilis

The treatment is the same as for primary syphilis if the cerebrospinal fluid (CSF) examination is negative. If a CSF exam is not done, benzathine penicillin G, 2.4 million units (1.2 million units in each buttock), should be given three or four times at one-week intervals for a total dose of 7.2–9.6 million units.

Late syphilis

Four doses of benzathine penicillin G, 2.4 million units, should be given at one-week intervals for a total dose of 9.6 million units. An alternative treatment is aqueous procaine penicillin G, 600,000 units intramuscularly daily, for a total dose of 9 million units.

Syphilis in pregnancy

Pregnant patients should be treated as soon as the diagnosis is made. Because of the probability that an intramuscular dose of benzathine penicillin G given to the mother will not cross the blood-brain barrier of the fetus, a pregnant woman should be treated with a course of aqueous procaine penicillin G. Although it was previously thought that syphilis does not cross the placenta before the eighteenth week of pregnancy, recent data [17] have shown the presence of spirochetes in two fetuses of only 9 and 10 weeks' gestation. Thus, it must be assumed that all pregnant women require effective therapy to cure syphilitic infection of the fetus, regardless of gestational age.

Congenital syphilis

If there is no central nervous system involvement, benzathine penicillin G, 50,000 units/kg intramuscularly, should be given. If no CSF exam is done or if it is positive, aqueous penicillin G, 50,000 units/kg intramuscularly, divided into two doses, should be given over 10 days.

ALTERNATE THERAPY FOR PENICILLIN-ALLERGIC PATIENTS

Primary or secondary syphilis

Treatment for primary or secondary syphilis in penicillin-allergic patients is tetracycline (or erythromycin), 24–40 gm given over 10–15 days (e.g., tetracycline 500 mg four times a day for 15 days).

Late syphilis

Treatment for late syphilis is tetracycline (or erythromycin), 60–80 gm total dosage.

Pregnant patients

Optimal therapy has not been established for penicillin-allergic pregnant patients with syphilis. Since tetracycline is probably contraindicated, the two options are erythromycin and the cephalosporins. The latter must be used with caution because of possible allergic reactions. If erythromycin is used, the dosage is the same as that given above for primary syphilis; if cephaloridine is used, the dosage is 0.5–1.0 gm intramuscularly for 10 days (this probably will be replaced with cefazolin sodium). Careful follow-up is required because of the lack of extensive evaluation of the alternative regimens.

FOLLOW-UP

Patients should be referred to the state Venereal Disease Clinic for follow-up. Serological tests are checked at regular intervals for one year in patients with primary or secondary syphilis and for two years in patients with latent or late syphilis. In most cases the test becomes negative in 6–12 months after treatment of primary syphilis and 12–24 months after treatment for secondary syphilis. If the serological tests remain positive, examination of the spinal fluid and retreatment is recommended [18]. The tests may remain positive indefinitely in patients with latent or late syphilis, thus necessitating at least yearly follow-up of quantitative serological tests to ensure that the titer is not increasing.

PREVENTION OF VENEREAL DISEASE

Careful screening of sexually active adolescents, follow-up of contacts, and easy access to treatment should help to prevent the epidemic spread of venereal diseases. Encouraging steady relationships and the use of condoms may also help. Education on venereal disease should be part of human sexuality courses in schools and churches; a dire warning of the consequences of venereal disease given in a one-hour school assembly is not likely to be helpful to teenagers. Specific facts, including local treatment centers, should be discussed; many teen-agers and doctors still feel that "nice girls don't get V.D.," and the diagnosis may therefore be missed.

REFERENCES

1. Ris, H. W., and Dodge, R. W. Gonorrhea in adolescent girls in a closed population. *Am. J. Dis. Child.* 123:185, 1972.
2. Litt, I., et al. Gonorrhea in children and adolescents. *J. Pediatr.* 85:595, 1974.
3. Keith, L., et al. Gonorrhea detection in a family planning clinic: A cost-benefit analysis of 2000 triplicate cultures. *Am. J. Obstet. Gynecol.* 121: 399, 1975.
4. Green, R. L., et al. Plasma procaine concentrations after procaine penicillin G. *N. Engl. J. Med.* 291:223, 1974.
5. Wiesner, P. J., et al. Clinical spectrum of pharyngeal gonococcal infection. *N. Engl. J. Med.* 288:181, 1973.
6. Lukasik, L. A. Comparative evaluation of the bacteriological flora of the uterine cervix and fallopian tubes in cases of salpingitis. *Am. J. Obstet. Gynecol.* 87:1028, 1963.
7. Eschenbach, D., et al. Polymicrobial etiology of acute pelvic inflammatory disease. *N. Engl. J. Med.* 293:166, 1975.
8. McCormick, W. M., et al. The genital mycoplasmas. *N. Engl. J. Med.* 288:78, 1973.
9. Jacobson, L. Laparoscopy in the diagnosis of acute salpingitis. *Acta Obstet. Gynecol. Scand.* 43:160, 1964.
10. Jacobson, L., and Westrom, L. Objectivized diagnosis of acute pelvic inflammatory disease. *Am. J. Obstet. Gynecol.* 105:1088, 1969.
11. Westrom, L. Effect of acute pelvic inflammatory disease on fertility. *Am. J. Obstet. Gynecol.* 121:707, 1975.
12. Holmes, K., et al. Disseminated gonococcal infection. *Ann. Intern. Med.* 74:979, 1971.
13. Keiser, H., et al. Clinical forms of gonococcal arthritis. *N. Engl. J. Med.* 279:234, 1968.
14. Blankership, R., et al. Treatment of disseminated gonococcal infection. *N. Engl. J. Med.* 290:267, 1974.
15. U.S. Public Health Service, Center for Disease Control. Gonorrhea: Recommended treatment schedules, 1974. *J. Pediatr.* 86:794, 1975.
16. Krugman, S., and Ward, R. *Infectious Diseases of Children and Adults.* Saint Louis: Mosby, 1973.
17. Harter, C., and Benirschke, K. Fetal syphilis in the first trimester. *Am. J. Obstet. Gynecol.* 124:705, 1976.
18. Fiumara, N. Venereal Diseases. In J. Gallagher, F. Heald, and D. Garell (Eds.), *Medical Care of the Adolescent* (3rd ed.). New York: Appleton-Century-Crofts, 1976.

10. In Utero Exposure to Diethylstilbestrol

During the 1950s and early 1960s diethylstilbestrol (DES) and other nonsteroidal estrogens were given to pregnant women with the intention of preventing miscarriages. In 1970 Herbst et al. [1] reported an association between maternal DES and the later development of clear cell adenocarcinoma of the vagina and cervix in female offspring. More recently adenosis, the presence of glandular (columnar) epithelium of müllerian origin in the vaginal wall (normally stratified squamous epithelium), has been described in 36 to 90 percent of exposed young women [2, 3, 4]. Although adenosis is a benign lesion, the proximity of areas of adenosis to adenocarcinoma in several patients has necessitated the follow-up of all patients with DES exposure.

PATIENT EVALUATION
The number of exposed young women is estimated to range from at least several hundred thousand to perhaps several million. Reliable histories are often difficult to obtain; thus *all* patients (prepubertal and postpubertal) who have abnormal bleeding or discharge should have a vaginal examination regardless of history. What should the general physician do?

1. Determine the maternal drug history on all patients.
2. Refer for gynecological exam at menarche or age 14 all patients with a known maternal history of any amount of DES or other nonsteroidal estrogen.
3. Be available for counseling and discussion of the importance of gynecological follow-up.

Point 3 is particularly important because it is not unusual for mothers to feel extremely guilty about having taken the medication; some ask to have their daughters checked under some other pretext. The adolescent girl may express great anger toward her mother for having made her body imperfect. However, in general it is much less destructive to a teenager to deal with these issues openly than to allow the doctor and mother to have a "secret." Although mothers and daughters are usually seeking reassurance that the vagina is "clean," the high frequency of adenosis indicates that this is not possible. Even though the carcinoma risk is minimal (probably less than 4/1000) [5], the long-term risk of the presence of adenosis is unknown.

123

The gynecological examination of the teenager exposed in utero to DES consists of:

1. Careful palpation of the vagina.
2. Speculum examination with Papanicolaou (Pap) smear and Schiller's stain of the vagina.
3. Biopsies as indicated by the Schiller's stain.

If colposcopy is available, follow-up is greatly facilitated. The colposcope is a binocular, low-power microscope that is used to examine the cervix and vagina with a speculum in place; the whole spectrum of atypia, dysplasia, and carcinoma can then be identified. Photographs can be taken and then reviewed at subsequent visits. Colposcopy detects more cases of adenosis (80–90 percent) than visual exam (less than 30 percent) or Schiller's stains (40–80 percent).

For those physicians interested in the actual statistics of adenocarcinoma and adenosis, a brief summary of recent work is given below and in the references at the end of this chapter.

INCIDENCE OF ADENOCARCINOMA AND ADENOSIS

ADENOCARCINOMA

Although sporadic cases of clear cell adenocarcinoma of the cervix and vagina had been reported prior to the 1960s, the incidence has risen dramatically since 1966. Of the 170 cases collected by Herbst et al. [6], information on maternal medication was obtained in 146 patients as noted below:

Stilbestrol, dienestrol, or hexestrol	84
One of the above and progestational agent	11
Hormone medication of unknown type for bleeding	19
Progestational agent alone	1
No history of above medications	31
	146

Herbst's data showed a wide range of dosage and duration of DES therapy; some mothers had an extremely short course of low dose DES. In all cases nonsteroidal estrogens were started prior to the eighteenth week of pregnancy.

At the time of diagnosis, most patients presented with bleeding or discharge, but 28 patients were asymptomatic. It is of great importance that, of the asymptomatic patients discovered to have cancer on routine examination done solely because of a positive maternal history, all are now living. The Pap smear can be helpful and was reported as positive or suspicious in 76 percent of cancer patients; in 11 patients, the Pap smear was the first clue to diagnosis. However,

125

it should be noted that 20 patients had a benign Pap smear, indicating that a normal report does not rule out adenocarcinoma of the vagina.

The average age of young women at the time of diagnosis was 17½ to 18 years; however, it is unclear whether the age will increase as time elapses or whether this represents the peak at risk. Occasional cases have occurred in prepubertal girls, but all had symptoms of bleeding for weeks to months prior to the diagnosis.

The current recommendation of Herbst et al. for therapy of stage I and stage II tumors is radical hysterectomy. Metastatic disease is common and implies a poor prognosis.

ADENOSIS

In contrast to the rare occurrence of adenocarcinoma, adenosis is a common finding in young women exposed in utero to DES; it is reported in 36–90 percent of patients. Adenosis is the presence of glandular epithelium of müllerian origin (similar to endocervix and endometrium) in the vaginal wall. Exposure to DES appears to have interfered with normal differentiation and development of the cervix and vagina. The wide range of reported cases of adenosis is in part related to the method of detection (colposcopy versus Schiller's stain) and in part related to lesions included. Most investigators include patients with an extensive congenital erosion that virtually covers the portio in the 90 percent figure. Several typical gross lesions have been de-

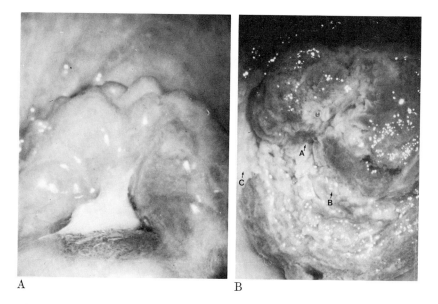

A   B

Fig. 10-1. Colposcopic view of cervix in patients exposed in utero to DES. (A) Cock's-comb appearance; (B) fibrous ridge (c) and extensive erosion (B) partially obscuring the cervical os (A).

Table 10-1. Results of Pelvic Examinations in Patients Exposed to DES Compared to Control Patients

Lesion	Patients Exposed to DES (Percent)	Control Patients
Nonstaining vagina	56	1
Nonstaining cervix	95	49
Adenosis	35	1[a]
Erosion	85	38
Vaginal or cervical fibrous ridges	22	0

[a] One case with inclusion cyst.
Source: Adapted from A. Herbst [7].

scribed, including (1) "vaginal hood"—a circular fold that partially covers the cervix, (2) "cock's-comb" appearance of the cervix—an irregular peak on the anterior border of the cervix, (3) erythroplakia—reddish areas that may give the cervix or vagina a "strawberry" appearance, and (4) fibrous ridges (Fig. 10-1).

Herbst et al. [7] studied two populations of young women in which the examiner was unaware whether the patient was exposed to DES or a control. The lesions noted have a striking incidence in the DES group (see Table 10-1).

The fact that adenosis is commonly found adjacent to foci of clear cell adenocarcinoma necessitates careful follow-up of this lesion. No form of treatment for adenosis has been determined, although there is some evidence that spontaneous healing occurs. Unless biopsies indicate atypical changes that necessitate local excision, the most prudent course appears to be follow-up examinations every six months and in some cases cryocautery.

REFERENCES

1. Herbst, A., et al. Adenocarcinoma of the vagina. N. Engl. J. Med. 284: 878, 1971.
2. Burke, L., et al. Vaginal adenosis: Correlation of colposcopic and pathologic findings. Obstet. Gynecol. 44:257, 1974.
3. Stafe, A., et al. Clinical diagnosis of vaginal adenosis. Obstet. Gynecol. 43:118, 1974.
4. Sherman, A. I., et al. Cervical-vaginal adenosis after in utero exposure to synthetic estrogens. Obstet. Gynecol. 44:531, 1974.
5. Lanier, A., et al. Cancer and stilbestrol: A follow-up of 1719 persons exposed to estrogens in utero and born 1943–1959. Mayo Clin. Proc. 48: 793, 1973.
6. Herbst, A., et al. Clear cell adenocarcinoma of the vagina and cervix: Analysis of 170 registry cases. Am. J. Obstet. Gynecol. 119:713, 1974.
7. Herbst, A. A prospective comparison of exposed female offspring with unexposed controls. N. Engl. J. Med. 292:334, 1975.

11. Ovarian Tumors

The scope of this book is not intended to include the histology and treatment of ovarian tumors in detail, because the general physician will only infrequently encounter such a tumor. Ovarian tumors are the most common genital neoplasms in childhood; however, overall ovarian tumors account for only about 1 percent of childhood tumors. Fortunately, most are benign.

DETECTION OF OVARIAN TUMORS

In the young child, an ovarian tumor is often accidentally discovered by the mother or physician as an asymptomatic abdominal mass because the pelvis is too small to contain an enlarging lesion for very long. Chronic aching abdominal pain, either periumbilical or located in one lower quadrant, is frequently present. Occasionally, acute severe pain, simulating acute appendicitis or peritonitis, may develop secondary to torsion, perforation, or infarction of a tumor. In some cases the patient may experience intermittent crampy pain, presumably on the basis of partial torsion, which subsequently resolves without therapy. Nonspecific symptoms including nausea, vomiting, a sense of abdominal fullness or bloating, and urinary frequency or retention may signal the presence of a tumor. In the young child, a granulosa cell tumor or an ovarian cyst may secrete estrogen, causing precocious development and menses; in the adolescent such tumors may be associated with hypermenorrhea and irregular periods.

The wide variety of possible symptoms suggests that the simplest method of detection is a bimanual rectal-abdominal (or rectal-vaginal-abdominal) examination in any patient with nonspecific abdominal complaints. In one large Boston study of ovarian tumors in adolescents (including cysts greater than 5 cm), 76 percent of the patients had a mass or tenderness on vaginal exam, 63 percent had a mass or tenderness on rectal exam, and 49 percent had a mass on abdominal exam [1]. Ovarian tumors should always be considered in the differential diagnosis of abdominal masses; the list of other possibilities is long and includes mesenteric cysts, hydronephrosis, liver cysts, bowel reduplication, Wilms' tumor, neuroblastoma, urachal cysts, and hematometra. A large, thin-walled cyst may be confused with ascites. A firm midline tumor in the adolescent may simulate a pregnant uterus. It should be remembered that the pregnancy test is positive in patients with choriocarcinoma and molar pregnancies (both rare in the adolescent). Small pelvic tumors in the sexually active teenager may occasionally be confused with an ectopic pregnancy or a hydrosalpinx (secondary to pelvic inflammatory disease [PID]). With an ectopic pregnancy, menstrual irregularities are common and the quantitative

urine pregnancy test may detect low levels of human chorionic gonadotropin (HCG). The serum β-subunit HCG, if available, is also positive.
In contrast, the patient with PID usually has bilateral tenderness, an
elevated sedimentation rate, and good response to antibiotic therapy.

Additional diagnostic procedures for a suspected ovarian tumor include a sonar scan, flat plate of the abdomen, intravenous pyelogram,
and possibly an arteriogram. Calcification is present on x-ray in approximately 40 percent of benign cystic teratomas. If the diagnosis
remains in doubt, laparoscopy or laparotomy is indicated.

CATEGORIES OF OVARIAN TUMORS

The majority of ovarian tumors are benign. Depending on the series,
10–38 percent are malignant. The major categories are listed below.
The incidence of simple cysts and benign teratomas is probably
higher than indicated because percentages are based on reported cases.
Treatment is discussed in the references [2–8]; with the exception of
cysts, referral to a large center is usually indicated.

GERM CELL TUMORS

Teratoma-dermoids account for about 30 percent of ovarian tumors
(the incidence ranges from 20–60 percent). Dermoids (80 percent of
this category) are cystic tumors composed predominantly of ecto-
dermal elements; 10–25 percent are bilateral. Teratomas (20 percent)
are solid tumors, composed of all three germ layers, and are malignant
in 25–50 percent of cases.

Dysgerminomas, which account for 3–7 percent of ovarian tumors,
tend to occur in childhood or late in life; approximately one-third are
malignant. This tumor is more common in patients with abnormalities
of the sex chromosomes. Five to ten percent of these tumors are
bilateral.

TUMORS OF EPITHELIAL AND STROMAL ORIGIN

Ten to twenty percent of ovarian tumors are cystadenomas, which
are epithelial tumors filled with pseudomucinous (pseudomucinous
cystadenomas) or cystic fluid (serous cystadenomas). Pseudomucinous
cystadenomas may undergo malignant degeneration in 10–14 percent
of cases.

GONADOBLASTOMAS

Gonadoblastomas (rare) are composed of germ cells and sex cord
cells. They occur most frequently in female patients with a "Y" line—
e.g., male pseudohermaphroditism (XY) or mixed gonadal dysgenesis
(XX/XY, XO/XY).

Sex Cord Mesenchyma Tumors

Granulosa theca cell tumors, which account for 3–5 percent of ovarian tumors, secrete estrogens and therefore may produce pseudoprecocious puberty in young girls and menstrual irregularities including hypermenorrhea in postmenarcheal adolescents. Approximately 3 percent are malignant.

Arrhenoblastomas (rare) are mixed Sertoli-Leydig cell tumors, which secrete androgens and thus produce heterosexual precocity in young children and virilization in adolescents. About 25 percent are malignant.

Sertoli cell tumors, which are also rare, may present as an abdominal mass or cause isosexual pseudoprecocious puberty in the young child.

Solid Ovarian Carcinoma

Although in some cases histology suggests that a solid ovarian carcinoma originated from a cystadenoma, in most cases these tumors show anaplasia that necessitates classification as an undifferentiated carcinoma. These tumors are highly malignant.

Functional Cysts

Functional cysts (20–50 percent of ovarian tumors) are not true tumors but rather should be considered a variation of the normal physiological process. In fact, it is not unusual to find small follicular cysts in the ovaries of healthy children and adolescents. Occasionally, after the oocyte dies, an atretic follicle may enlarge to 6–8 cm in diameter, producing a follicular cyst. In young children, a hormone-secreting cyst may cause sexual precocity. Rarely large cysts are found in neonates secondary to in utero stimulation by maternal gonadotropins; more commonly these cysts occur in the postmenarcheal adolescent.

In some cases, menstrual irregularity or pain (secondary to torsion or rupture) brings the patient to the physician. In many cases, follicular cysts are found on routine examination and resolve spontaneously in one to two months. If a small cyst is palpated in an asymptomatic patient, oral contraceptive pills may be prescribed to suppress the hypothalamic-ovarian axis; the patient should be examined monthly. If the mass has not resolved within three months or is large on initial examination, laparoscopy is indicated. The fluid can be aspirated from the cyst during this procedure.

Corpus luteum cysts are less common than follicular cysts and may reach 5–10 cm in diameter. Although such cysts are often asymptomatic, they may cause amenorrhea (secondary to continued production of progesterone and estrogen) and then profuse vaginal bleeding as the cyst becomes atretic. Occasionally, these cysts are responsible for crampy lower abdominal pain caused by torsion or hemorrhage; in fact, rupture of the blood-filled cyst can precipitate an acute abdominal emergency. In the absence of pain or intraperitoneal bleeding, therapy with oral contraceptive pills and observation for three months is indicated. If hemorrhage or pain occurs or the cyst is large on initial examination, laparoscopy or laparotomy is clearly necessary.

REFERENCES

1. Heald, F. Ovarian Tumors in Adolescence. In Heald, F. (Ed.), *Adolescent Gynecology*. Baltimore: Williams & Wilkins, 1966.
2. Smith, J., et al. Malignant gynecologic tumors in children: Current approaches to treatment. *Am. J. Obstet. Gynecol.* 116:261, 1973.
3. Huffman, J. *The Gynecology of Childhood and Adolescence*. Philadelphia: Saunders, 1969.
4. Green, T. *Gynecology: Essentials of Clinical Practice* (3rd ed.). Boston: Little, Brown, 1977.
5. Abell, M., et al. Ovarian neoplasms in childhood: Tumors of germ cell origin. *Am. J. Obstet. Gynecol.* 92:1059, 1965.
6. Abell, M., et al. Ovarian neoplasms in childhood and adolescence: Tumors of non-germ cell origin. *Am. J. Obstet. Gynecol.* 93:850, 1965.
7. Ein, S., et al. Cystic and solid ovarian tumors in children: A forty-four year review. *J. Pediatr. Surg.* 5:148, 1970.
8. Nielsen, O. Ovarian tumors in children. *Acta Obstet. Gynecol. Scand.* 47:119, 1968.

12. The Breast: Examination and Lesions

Between the ages of 9 and 14, the majority of girls begin their adolescent breast development. Because breast development is often regarded as the principal sign of feminine sexuality, mothers and teenagers often worry inordinately about minor asymmetry or "inadequate" development. It is often difficult for the teenager to accept small breasts as "normal." On the other hand, reassurance is in order only if the remainder of the examination and history excludes an endocrine disorder. Recent national publicity on breast cancer has made adolescents exceptionally anxious about cystic changes and fibroadenomas. Perhaps this fear can be utilized constructively to encourage patients to begin monthly self-examinations.

BREAST EXAMINATION

All patients should have a careful breast examination regardless of whether specific complaints are mentioned. The patient is first asked to sit facing the examiner, and the breasts are inspected for asymmetry, retraction of the nipple, and dimpling of the skin. The patient is then asked to lie supine with her arm extended over her head. Breast development should be recorded as Tanner stages B1–B5 (see Chap. 4). If asymmetry or disorders of development are a concern, then exact measurement of the areola and breast should be included at each exam (Fig. 12–1).

For example, one might record the following:

	Areola	Breast
Right	2.5 cm	8 × 9 cm
Left	2.5 cm	9 × 10 cm

The first number in the breast figure is the upper to lower measurement; the second number is the right to left measurement. The breast tissue should be carefully palpated in a straight line laterally, clockwise around the breast (Fig. 12-2). The flat portion of the fingers should be moved in a slightly rotatory fashion to feel abnormal masses. Normal glandular tissue has an irregular, granular surface like tapioca pudding. In contrast, a fibroadenoma feels firm and smooth. The areola should be gently compressed to assess any abnormal discharge. During the exam the physician should instruct the teenager in self-examination to be done after each menstrual period.

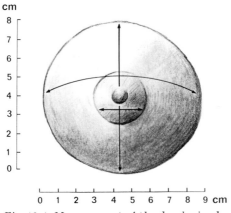

Fig. 12-1. Measurement of the developing breast.

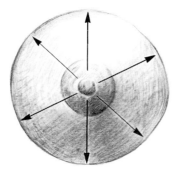

Fig. 12-2. Palpation of the breast: the fingers are moved in a straight line laterally around the breast.

PROBLEMS OF BREAST DEVELOPMENT

ASYMMETRY

Asymmetry of the breasts is a very common complaint, especially during the early stages of development. Since the breast bud may initially appear on one side as a tender, granular lump, mothers are often concerned about the possibility of a tumor. Reassurance and observation are in order. Asymmetry during development may be treated with a brassiere pad for the smaller breast. A major difference can be treated with a foam insert (available in department stores for mastectomy patients). In certain patients a mammoplasty may be considered after full development is attained (Fig. 12–3).

The possibility of a giant fibroadenoma should always be excluded by physical examination. Such fibroadenomas are usually solitary, and the overlying skin is typically taut with dilatation of the superficial veins.

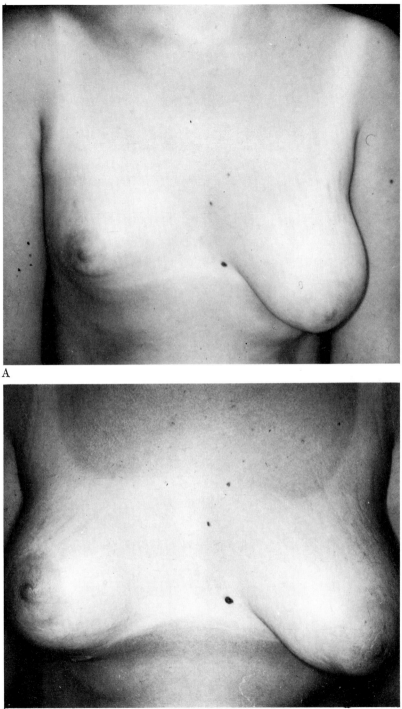

A

B

Fig. 12-3. Sixteen-year-old girl with hypoplasia of the right breast. (A) Pre-operatively, (B) after augmentation mammoplasty with a Cronin prosthesis. (Courtesy of George E. Gifford, M.D., Children's Hospital, Boston.)

HYPERTROPHY

True hypertrophy of the breast(s) occasionally occurs during adolescence. Instead of ceasing to enlarge at the normal limits, the breast(s) continues to increase in size (Fig. 12-4). The menstrual history is usually normal; the etiology of this problem has not been defined. Mayl et al. [1] recently reported the successful use of dydrogesterone (Gynorest), a progestational agent, in four patients with actively enlarging breasts. They recommended that surgical reduction be delayed if possible until growth had ceased.

LACK OF DEVELOPMENT

Lack of development may be secondary to congenital absence of glandular tissue (amastia) or to a systemic disorder, e.g., malnutrition (including Crohn's disease), congenital adrenal hyperplasia, gonadal dysgenesis, or hypogonadotropic hypogonadism. The evaluation depends on the history and physical findings. Normal sexual hair development and regular periods would suggest congenital amastia. Amenorrhea and oligomenorrhea require a thorough investigation, as discussed in Chapter 6.

PREMATURE THELARCHE

A discussion of premature thelarche can be found in Chapter 5.

ACCESSORY NIPPLES OR BREASTS

Accessory nipples or breasts occur in 1–2 percent of healthy patients. In some cases all three components of the breast—glandular tissue, areola, and nipple—are present. More commonly only a small areola and nipple are found, usually along the embryological milk line between the axillae and groin. No therapy is necessary. Engorgement of accessory breasts is common during pregnancy and lactation. If no outlet is present, the breast tissue spontaneously involutes within several days to weeks after delivery.

NIPPLE DISCHARGE

Nipple discharge is a rare problem. Postpartum and postabortion women may have galactorrhea (a thin, milky discharge) for a year or more. Galactorrhea occasionally occurs in patients taking phenothiazines, reserpine, methyldopa, and oral contraceptive pills. It has also been associated with hypothyroidism, adrenal disorders, and surgery or trauma to the chest wall. A history of amenorrhea in addition to galactorrhea necessitates an evaluation to exclude a central nervous system tumor. The finding of a blood-tinged discharge should prompt a search for an intraductal papilloma or carcinoma.

Occasionally a periareolar follicle will drain a small amount of brownish fluid for several weeks; no treatment is usually necessary.

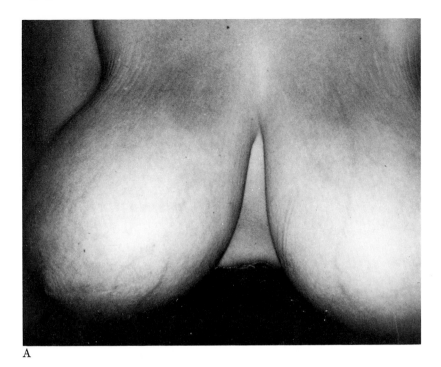

A

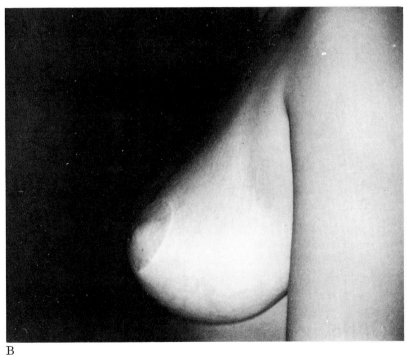

B

Fig. 12-4. Nineteen-year-old woman with virginal hypertrophy of both breasts, resulting in back pain and a dorsal kyphosis. (A) Preoperatively, (B) after reduction mammoplasty. (Courtesy of George E. Gifford, M.D., Children's Hospital, Boston.)

Periareolar Hair

Periareolar hair is not uncommon in the healthy adolescent. Cosmetic treatment (usually unnecessary) can be accomplished by plucking, which is painful, or by cutting the hairs.

BREAST MASSES

Fibrocystic Disease versus Fibroadenoma

Fibrocystic disease is probably responsible for most breast masses in the adolescent. In the typical patient, the breasts have diffuse, cordlike thickenings and lumps which may become tender and enlarged prior to each menses. Physical findings tend to change each month, so the suspected cyst can often be followed carefully. It is important to encourage the teenager to become aware of her cysts by monthly self-examination.

In contrast, a fibroadenoma is usually firm or rubbery and either remains unchanged or increases in size with subsequent examination. Recurrent or multiple fibroadenomas are not uncommon.

If an abnormal mass is palpated, the adolescent should be instructed to return after her next period. If the lesion has disappeared, a cyst was probably present. If the lesion remains unchanged or has increased in size, aspiration can be done with a 21-gauge needle attached to a 10-cc syringe. Any material obtained (even if just on the tip of the needle) should be smeared on a ground glass slide and sent in Papanicolaou's fixative for cytology examination. If no fluid is present, a fibroadenoma may be present, and the patient should be referred for excision. Since breast scars can be cosmetically deforming, the optimal incision for a lesion near the center of the breast is a circumareolar incision. Such procedures can usually be done in an ambulatory setting under general or local anesthesia. Follow-up is important because of the recurrent nature of cysts and fibroadenomas.

Contusion

A contusion to the breast may result in a poorly defined, tender mass that resolves over several weeks. A mass from severe trauma may take several months to resolve, and occasionally scar tissue remains palpable indefinitely. Fat necrosis may also result from trauma, although the patient may not notice the growing lesion until several months later. Biopsy is frequently indicated in such circumstances. It should be remembered that the examination immediately following trauma to the breast may locate a preexisting lesion. A sharply delineated, nontender mass is probably unrelated to the recent injury.

Infection

Infection of the breast is uncommon except in newborns and lactating women. Usually the history includes the sudden onset of a warm, tender mass with redness of the overlying skin. Staphylococci are the most common pathogens, although gram-negative organisms may cause infection in the newborn. Most cases of mastitis respond to systemic antibiotics and incision and drainage (if the mass becomes fluctuant). The recurrence rate is high for subareolar abscesses in adults [2].

CARCINOMA

Cancer of the breast is extremely rare in children and adolescents [3, 4, 5]. Of all patients reported by Haagensen [6] with breast cancer, only 0.2 percent were less than 25 years old. In a series of 237 patients (10 to 20 years old) with breast lesions, Farrow and Ashikari [7] reported only one patient with primary breast carcinoma and two patients with sarcomas metastatic to breast tissue. Cystosarcoma phylloides is a rare primary breast tumor that is occasionally malignant. Nevertheless, all breast lesions excised should be sent for pathological examination, and young women with a strong family history of breast cancer should have careful follow-up.

REFERENCES

1. Mayl, N., et al. Treatment of macromastia in the actively enlarging breast. *Plast. Reconstr. Surg.* 54:6, 1974.
2. Ekland, D., and Zeigler, M. Abscess in the nonlactating breast. *Arch. Surg.* 107:398, 1973.
3. Daniel, W., and Matthews, M. Tumors of the breast in adolescent females. *Pediatrics* 41:743, 1968.
4. Oberman, H., and Stephens, P. Carcinoma of the breast in childhood. *Cancer* 30:470, 1972.
5. Simpson, L., and Barson, A. Breast tumors in infants and children. *Can. Med. Assoc. J.* 101:100, 1969.
6. Haagensen, C. D. *Diseases of the Breast* (2nd ed.). Philadelphia: Saunders, 1971.
7. Farrow, J., and Ashikari, H. Breast lesions in young girls. *Surg. Clin. North Am.* 49:261, 1969.

SELECTED READING

Sandison, A., and Welker, J. Diseases of the adolescent female breast. *Br. J. Surg.* 55:443, 1968.
Schauffler, G. *Pediatric Gynecology.* Chicago: Year Book, 1958.
Turbey, W., et al. The surgical management of pediatric breast masses. *Pediatrics* 56:736, 1975.

13. Hirsutism

The physician is sometimes faced with the evaluation of the young girl or teenager with hirsutism. In most cases, the etiology is related to familial or racial factors; the explanation seems to rest in the varying capacity of the hair follicle to respond to different androgen levels, perhaps in a genetically determined way. In some cases, ovarian or adrenal androgen production is found to be excessive; thus, it is always appropriate to give the problem careful consideration before dismissing it. Whatever the cause, the patient may still benefit from hints on therapy. If she has the courage to bring up the subject, she deserves the time to discuss it.

DEFINING HIRSUTISM

Two types of hair are found on the human body: terminal hair (greater than 0.5 cm in length, coarse, and usually pigmented) and vellus or lanugo (downy, fine, light-colored hair). An increase in the distribution and quantity of terminal hair may bring the patient to the physician with the complaint of hirsutism. Excessive downy hair is usually referred to as *hypertrichosis*. Difficulty arises, of course, in establishing whether the amount of hair is excessive, since the spectrum of "normal" is at best ill defined.

McKnight [1] studied 400 normal young women in Wales in an attempt to establish the prevalence of terminal hair. She found that the great majority of women had terminal hair on the lower arm and leg (84 percent) and most also had terminal hair on the upper arm and leg (70 percent). Twenty-six percent had terminal hair on the face, usually on the upper lip. In 10 percent of the women, the facial hair was noticeable, and in 4 percent it was characterized as a "true disfigurement." Seventeen percent had hair on the chest or breast, usually periareolar; 35 percent had hair on the abdomen, usually along the linea alba up to the umbilicus; 16 percent had hair in the lumbosacral area; and 3 percent had hair on the upper back. Nine percent had considerable hair in most or all of these areas and were, therefore, considered "hirsute."

A number of recent studies have emphasized the relation of serum androgen to hirsutism, but results have been variable and the samples small. For example, Rosenfeld [2] found that 35 percent of 20 hirsute patients had an elevated plasma testosterone, and an additional 25 percent had a normal (total) testosterone with an elevated free testosterone level (testosterone binding globulin was decreased). Abraham [3] reported that 82 percent of his 17 hirsute patients had elevated testosterone and 90 percent had increased 17-hydroxyproges-terone levels. Further studies to delineate the adrenal and ovarian contributions to the excess androgens are underway [4, 5]. These studies are intriguing, and perhaps in the future sophisticated tests will become available to the clinician to evaluate and treat the problem of hirsutism. At the present time, however, the study of most hirsute patients should conform to the following guidelines.

PATIENT EVALUATION

What approach should the general physician take? First, the history should focus on (1) recent change in the amount of hair, (2) location of new hair, and (3) relation of hair development to the onset of puberty and menses. Increased hair, especially if coarse, over the face, chest, abdomen, or back is usually significant. Hirsutism associated with menstrual irregularity deserves careful attention.

The physical examination should include notation of the distribution and quality of the hair and the presence of any signs of virilization—temporal hair recession, deepening of the voice, clitoral enlargement, or changes in body fat and muscle distribution. A vaginal or rectal examination should be done to assess ovarian size if the patient has significant hirsutism, signs of virilization, or irregular menstrual periods.

Most patients with mild hirsutism and regular periods will have a familial or racial predisposition. Other less common causes of mild hirsutism include exogenous medication (e.g., diphenylhydantoin, prednisone, diazoxide, androgens), the Stein-Leventhal syndrome (see p. 91), pregnancy, hypothyroidism (usually associated with hypertrichosis), and chronic illness (e.g., mental and motor retardation, anorexia nervosa).

The patient with significant or progressive hirsutism, with or without virilization, requires a careful evaluation to try to establish a definitive diagnosis. Although in some patients both the adrenal glands and the ovaries contribute to the production of excess androgens, it is possible in many cases to define the source in terms of (1) gonads, (2) adrenal glands, or (3) iatrogenic causes. The term *gonad* is used because a small number of hirsute patients will have testicular tissue as the cause of virilization. The gonadal etiologies for hirsutism and/or virilization include the Stein-Leventhal syndrome (most common), ovarian hyperthecosis (hyperplastic theca cells in noncystic ovaries) [6], ovarian tumors, gonadal dysgenesis (XO) with virilization, mixed gonadal dysgenesis, and incomplete testicular feminization; these diagnoses are discussed in detail in Chapter 6. The adrenal gland may be the source of excess androgen secretion in patients with congenital (or adult-onset) adrenocortical hyperplasia (CAH), Cushing's syndrome, or adrenal tumors. As has already been discussed in Chapter 6, CAH may not be diagnosed in patients with a mild deficiency of 11 β-hydroxylase or 21-hydroxylase until hirsutism or oligomenorrhea

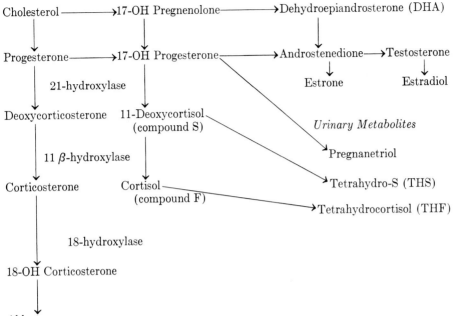

Fig. 13-1. Major pathways of steroid biosynthesis.

becomes evident in the teenage years. Iatrogenic causes are chiefly limited to the use of androgenic hormones in the treatment of hematological disorders.

The initial evaluation of the young woman with significant hirsutism should include (1) physical examination including a pelvic exam, (2) 24-hour urine test for 17-ketosteroids and 17-hydroxycorticosteroids, and (3) serum testosterone level. Further laboratory tests depend chiefly on the clinical assessment and the values of urinary 17-ketosteroids. A dexamethasone suppression test is essential in patients with elevated 17-ketosteroids. Other tests include a serum follicle-stimulating hormone (FSH), luteinizing hormone (LH), and 17-hydroxyprogesterone; buccal smear with Y fluorescence (and/or karyotype); and possibly laparoscopy. A review of the pathways of steroid synthesis and the urinary metabolites is shown in Figure 13-1; normal values for 17-ketosteroids are included in Appendix 1.

If the urinary 17-ketosteroids are mildly elevated (15–25 mg/24 hours), the patient most likely has either the Stein-Leventhal syndrome, ovarian hyperthecosis, or a mild form of congenital (or adult-onset) adrenocortical hyperplasia. A dexamethasone suppression test (0.5 mg every 6 hours for four days) will usually suppress 17-ketosteroids to 3–4 mg/24 hours in patients with adrenal disease and to

5–11 mg/24 hours in patients with ovarian disease. Occasionally, patients with adrenal disease may require either 0.5 mg every 6 hours for two weeks or 2 mg every 6 hours for three days for complete suppression. However, in some cases, the dexamethasone suppression test may not definitely distinguish between an ovarian and adrenal source for the excess androgens. In fact, recent data [7] suggest that in many hirsute patients the elevated testosterone production rates are suppressible by dexamethasone despite the ovarian source. If a research laboratory is available, the site of the partial block in adrenocorticoid synthesis (CAH) can be further elucidated by measurement of dehydroepiandrosterone, Tetrahydro-S, and pregnanetriol before and after infusion of adrenocorticotropic hormone. Elevated 17-hydroxycorticosteroids in a fat, hypertensive patient should prompt further evaluation to rule out Cushing's disease.

In patients with partial suppression of 17-ketosteroids by dexamethasone therapy, the Stein-Leventhal syndrome or ovarian hyperthecosis are likely possibilities. Serum testosterone may be normal or elevated. Confirmatory evidence of the diagnosis of polycystic ovaries is provided by the physical examination, LH levels that are often consistently above 30 mIU/ml (a tonic rather than cyclic secretion of LH) with normal FSH levels, and most significantly by laparoscopy and ovarian biopsy.

Patients with urinary 17-ketosteroids in excess of 25 mg/24 hours should also have a dexamethasone suppression test. If the elevated 17-ketosteroids are not suppressible, the patient must be evaluated for an adrenal or ovarian tumor.

If the 17-ketosteroids are normal in spite of virilization, a serum 17-hydroxyprogesterone and testosterone should be measured. An elevated serum testosterone indicates the presence of (1) polycystic ovaries of the Stein-Leventhal syndrome or ovarian hyperthecosis (most common), (2) a virilizing tumor, or (3) a functioning testis (mixed gonadal dysgenesis or male pseudohermaphroditism). A buccal smear with positive Y fluorescence suggests the third diagnosis; laparoscopy is often necessary to differentiate between the first two possibilities. Suppression of the polycystic ovaries with birth control pills should lower the serum testosterone; the same therapy in a patient with a tumor (although clearly not recommended) would in most cases not alter the testosterone value. Only a few cases of LH-dependent tumors have been reported thus far [8, 9]. Thus, a serum testosterone level done before and after one to two months on the pill would probably exclude the rare virilizing ovarian tumor.

It should be noted that hirsute patients with the Stein-Leventhal syndrome or ovarian hyperthecosis may have a normal testosterone value; presumably, an elevated free testosterone (serum values measure total testosterone), an increased testosterone secretion rate, or another androgen is responsible for the progressive hirsutism. Thus measurement of testosterone-binding globulin, unbound testosterone, and androstenedione in conjunction with laparoscopy may be indicated in patients with irregular periods and unexplained progressive hirsutism or virilization.

TREATMENT

Treatment of hirsutism consists of:

1. Treatment of the cause, if possible. Patients with congenital (or adult-onset) adrenocortical hyperplasia should receive glucocorticoid replacement as indicated on p. 86. Those with the Stein-Leventhal syndrome and hirsutism should be cycled with oral contraceptive pills (see p. 92). Thus far Ortho-Novum or Norinyl 2 mg and Ovral have been shown to be effective in suppressing plasma androstenedione and testosterone levels in approximately 80 percent of hirsute women [10]. One recent study [11] indicates that Ortho-Novum or Norinyl 1/80 decreases the unbound testosterone level but actually increases the total testosterone level by increasing testosterone-binding globulin. Our limited data have demonstrated a lowering of total testosterone with Ortho-Novum or Norinyl 1/50. In view of these inconsistencies, further experience is necessary to establish the optimal oral contraceptive for this purpose.

In patients with mixed gonadal dysgenesis or male pseudohermaphroditism removal of the dysgenetic testis(es) is necessary to prevent further virilization and possible malignant degeneration of the gonad. Virilizing tumors should be surgically resected, if possible. Unfortunately, in all of these conditions, treatment usually results only in partial regression of the hirsutism. The patient can at least be told that no new hair should grow and that therapy is possible to help with the removal of unwanted hair. Unless the patient is forewarned, disappointment may be followed by depression. In contrast, excess hair growth associated with pregnancy, hypothyroidism, or anorexia nervosa is usually reversible.

2. Bleaching and removal of the hair. Regardless of whether the source of the hirsutism is familial or organic, the patient needs help to achieve good cosmetic results. Bleaching of the fine hair, the first choice therapy, is accomplished with 6% hydrogen peroxide; the addition of 10 drops of ammonia per 30 cc of peroxide just before use will activate the peroxide and increase bleaching. Depilatories, shaving, and wax epilation remove hair temporarily. Electrolysis, if done by an experienced person, permanently destroys the hair bulb and in most cases avoids pitlike scars and regrowth of incompletely destroyed hairs [12].

REFERENCES

1. McKnight, E.   The prevalence of "hirsutism" in young women. *Lancet* 1:410, 1964.
2. Rosenfeld, R.   Plasma testosterone binding globulin and indexes of the concentration of unbound plasma androgen in normal and hirsute subjects. *J. Clin. Endocrinol. Metab.* 32:717, 1971.
3. Abraham, G., and Chakmakjian, Z.   Plasma steroids in hirsutism. *Obstet. Gynecol.* 44:171, 1974.
4. Abraham, G.   Ovarian and adrenal contribution to peripheral steroids during the menstrual cycle in two hirsute women. *Obstet. Gynecol.* 46:29, 1975.
5. Abraham, G., et al.   Ovarian and adrenal contribution to peripheral androgens in hirsute women. *Obstet. Gynecol.* 46:169, 1975.
6. Wentz, A., et al.   Ovarian hyperthecosis in the adolescent patient. *J. Pediatr.* 88:488, 1976.
7. Kirschner, M., et al.   Idiopathic hirsutism: An ovarian abnormality. *N. Engl. J. Med.* 294:637, 1976.
8. Givens, J., et al.   Remission of Acanthosis Nigricans associated with polycystic ovarian disease and a stromal luteoma. *J. Clin. Endocrinol. Metab.* 38:126, 1974.
9. Givens, J., et al.   A gonadotropin-responsive adrenocortical adenoma. *J. Clin. Endocrinol. Metab.* 38:126, 1974.
10. Givens, J., et al.   The effectiveness of two oral contraceptives in suppressing plasma androstenedione, testosterone, LH, and FSH, and in stimulating plasma testosterone-binding capacity in hirsute women. *Am. J. Obstet. Gynecol.* 124:333, 1976.
11. Easterling, W., et al.   Serum testosterone levels in the polycystic ovary syndrome. *Am. J. Obstet. Gynecol.* 120:385, 1974.
12. Arndt, K.   *Manual of Dermatologic Therapeutics.* Boston: Little, Brown, 1974.

SUGGESTED READING

Huffman, J.   *The Gynecology of Childhood and Adolescence.* Philadelphia: Saunders, 1969.
Leng, J., and Greenblatt, R.   Hirsutism in adolescent girls. *Pediatr. Clin. North Am.* 19(3):681, 1972.

14. Birth Control

Whether or not a physician ethically believes in the appropriateness of premarital sexual relations, the fact remains that teenagers are engaging in intercourse at younger and younger ages, most without any form of contraception. Rarely will a teenager of 14 or 15 years of age request contraceptives from a doctor unless she is specifically questioned about menstrual periods and sexual history; the college student of 18 or 19 is more likely to seek gynecological care on her own. The physician is often faced with a dilemma in providing care to the adolescent patient: To give contraception without any discussion implies approval of a particular form of behavior; to deny contraception sets up the physician to be the harsh parent figure who can later be blamed for an unwanted pregnancy.

Who should prescribe contraception depends on the physician's familiarity with routine pelvic examinations and his or her knowledge of the indications and contraindications for using the birth control pill, intrauterine device (IUD), and other methods. Many practicing physicians will probably choose to refer their patients to an obstetrician-gynecologist; it is hoped that in the future primary care doctors will gain sufficient experience in medical school and residency to give routine gynecological care to adolescents. If a referral is made, it is important to ascertain that the gynecologist is sympathetic in dealing with adolescents and that he or she is not prejudiced against certain methods (e.g., the IUD). In any case, knowledge of the efficacy and side effects of the various methods is essential in patient care. Several states have passed laws specifically allowing minors to give their own informed consent for birth control; although there have been no legal opinions against doctors prescribing contraceptives, this decision clearly depends on the family and the community.

The pregnancy rates of 100 women using different contraceptives for one year are listed in Table 14-1. For some teenagers, the pregnancy rate with the pill may climb to 9 pregnancies/100 woman-years because of missed pills and misunderstanding of the directions. Generally for good compliance teenagers need to obtain contraceptive advice within the framework of comprehensive health care [3]. The teenager must feel that she has actively participated in the decision on the best method of contraception for her life-style; the dialogue between physician and patient is of supreme importance.

ORAL CONTRACEPTIVE PILLS

Most teenagers choose oral contraceptive pills because of the low failure rate and relief from dysmenorrhea. The common pills and their hormonal content are listed in Table 14-2. The combination pills are

Table 14-1. Pregnancy Rates per 100 Woman-Years of Use with Different Contraceptives[a]

Type of Contraceptive	Theoretical Rate	Rate with Actual Use
Oral contraceptives		
Combination	0.1	0.7
Sequential[b]	0.5	1.4
Mini-pill	. . . .	1.5–3.0
IUDs		
Lippes Loop B	. . . .	7
Lippes Loop D	. . . .	2.7
Copper 7 (CU-7)	. . . .	1.1–2.5
Condom	2.6	3–20
Diaphragm with contraceptive jelly	. . . .	3–20
Vaginal foam	. . . .	28–35
Depo-Provera	. . . .	0.3

[a] Data from references 1, 2, 4, 32, and 40.
[b] Withdrawn from the market February 26, 1976.

the most frequently prescribed oral contraceptive agents. The combination pills prevent pregnancy by suppressing the ovarian-hypothalamic axis and thus ovulation; in addition they alter the endometrium to make implantation unlikely and increase the viscosity of the cervical mucus [5]. Selection of a particular pill depends on the patient's needs and her response. Some pills are estrogen dominant, others are progestin dominant; Figure 14-1 is an approximation of

Estrogen Dominant	Progestin Dominant

Enovid-E

  Ovulen

    Ortho-Novum 2 mg

      Ortho-Novum 1/80

        Demulen

          Ortho-Novum 1/50

            Ovral

              Norlestrin 2.5 mg

Fig. 14-1. The relative estrogen-progestin balance of some commonly used oral contraceptive pills.

Table 14-2. The Hormonal Content of Commonly Used
Oral Contraceptive Pills

Product	Estrogen	Progestin
Combination pills		
Enovid-E	Mestranol 0.1 mg	Norethynodrel 2.5 mg
Enovid 5 mg	Mestranol 0.075 mg	Norethynodrel 5 mg
Ortho-Novum 1/50, Norinyl 1/50	Mestranol 0.05 mg	Norethindrone 1 mg
Ortho-Novum 1/80, Norinyl 1/80	Mestranol 0.08 mg	Norethindrone 1 mg
Ortho-Novum 2 mg, Norinyl 2 mg	Mestranol 0.1 mg	Norethindrone 2 mg
Norlestrin 1 mg, Zorane 1/50	Ethinyl estradiol 0.05 mg	Norethindrone acetate 1 mg
Norlestrin 2.5 mg	Ethinyl estradiol 0.05 mg	Norethindrone acetate 2.5 mg
Ovulen	Mestranol 0.1 mg	Ethynodiol diacetate 1 mg
Demulen	Ethinyl estradiol 0.05 mg	Ethynodiol diacetate 1 mg
Ovral	Ethinyl estradiol 0.05 mg	Norgestrel 0.5 mg
Ovcon-50	Ethinyl estradiol 0.05 mg	Norethindrone 1 mg
Ovcon-35	Ethinyl estradiol 0.035 mg	Norethindrone 0.4 mg
Zorane 1.5/30, Loestrin 1.5/30	Ethinyl estradiol 0.03 mg	Norethindrone 1 mg
Zorane 1/20, Loestrin 1/20	Ethinyl estradiol 0.02 mg	Norethindrone 1 mg
Brevicon	Ethinyl estradiol 0.035 mg	Norethindrone 0.5 mg
Lo-Ovral	Ethinyl estradiol 0.03 mg	Norgestrel 0.3 mg
Sequential pills[a]		
Oracon	16 white: ethinyl estradiol 0.1 mg 6 pink: 25 mg dimethisterone, 0.1 mg ethinyl estradiol	
Ortho-Novum SQ	14 white: 0.08 mg mestranol 6 blue: 2 mg norethindrone, 0.08 mg mestranol	
Mini-pills		
Nor-Q.D. & Micronor		Norethindrone 0.35 mg
Ovrette		Norgestrel 0.075 mg

[a] Withdrawn from the market February 26, 1976.

the effects of these pills. The indications for selecting an estrogen-dominant pill are:

1. Hirsutism or acne
2. Premenopausal symptoms
3. Scanty periods (while on or off the pill)
4. Increased appetite and weight gain while on the pill
5. Alopecia
6. Moniliasis
7. Early-cycle spotting while on the pill

The indications for selecting a progestin-dominant pill are:

1. Mucorrhea
2. Cervical erosion
3. History of nausea or bloating while on the pill or with pregnancy
4. Fibroids
5. Fibrocystic breast disease
6. Cyclic premenstrual weight gain
7. Premenstrual tension
8. Dysmenorrhea
9. Hypermenorrhea
10. Late-cycle spotting while on the pill

The side effects and contraindications of oral contraceptives must be carefully understood before the pill is prescribed [6].

Side Effects and Contraindications

Nausea, bloating, and weight gain

In general, fluid retention is an estrogenic side effect, and increased appetite is probably secondary to the progestin. Most teenagers tolerate the middle-range pills—Ortho-Novum 1/50, Norinyl 1/50, Demulen, or Ovral—without difficulty. If fluid retention is a problem, a less estrogenic pill (such as Lo-Ovral, Zorane or Loestrin 1.5/30 or 1/20) may be tried, although breakthrough bleeding may be a troublesome side effect.

Breakthrough Bleeding

Breakthrough bleeding is the occurrence of vaginal bleeding while the patient is taking hormone tablets. Although early-cycle spotting is said to be related to estrogen deficiency and late-cycle spotting to progestin deficiency, a direct correlation is not always possible. Breakthrough bleeding often decreases with subsequent cycles on the same pill. If not, increasing the estrogen content of the pill will usually alleviate the problem; occasionally a change to a more progestational pill such as Ovral or Ortho-Novum 2 mg is helpful.

Headaches

The risk of the pill in patients with migraine is unknown, but caution is obviously indicated. Many patients do experience an increase in the number and severity of headaches while taking the pill. Decreasing the estrogen content in the pill may alleviate the situation; however, if headaches persist, changing to the mini-pill or another form of contraception may be the only solution.

Hypertension

The pill is not recommended in patients with hypertension. Approximately 5–7 percent of normotensive individuals develop hypertension (> 140/90) within weeks to several months of starting the pill [4, 7, 8, 9]. A familial predisposition may be involved. Oral contraceptive pills increase plasma renin substrate, renin activity, angiotensin, and aldosterone. Some studies [10, 11] have suggested that renin concentration falls in normotensive women because the elevated aldosterone levels prevent the release of renin from the juxtaglomerular cells. Women who develop hypertension show normal or elevated renin levels, suggesting an inadequate feedback response. This explanation does not fit all patients; another recent study [12] has suggested that some hypertensive patients may have inadequate inactivation of angiotensin.

An elevated blood pressure usually returns to normal within two weeks to three months (occasionally six months) after the pill is discontinued. Another form of contraception must be prescribed. Some of these patients may later develop sustained hypertension off the pill, suggesting a predisposition. Although it is perhaps a coincidence, several of our patients with contraceptive-induced hypertension have had either an asymptomatic urinary tract infection or renal anomalies; thus, a urine culture and an intravenous pyelogram are probably indicated even though the blood pressure has returned to normal.

Thrombophlebitis

The risk of developing deep vein thrombosis, pulmonary embolism, or cerebral thrombosis is increased about five to six times by the use of oral contraceptives. The mortality is nevertheless much less than with pregnancy, although pill-users are presumably selected from a healthy population.

Women ages 20–34   22.8/100,000 die from pregnancy
                     1.5/100,000 die from the pill

Except for Enovid, the risk of thrombophlebitis appears to rise with increasing estrogen dosage [13, 14, 15].

The pill is contraindicated in patients with a past history of thrombophlebitis, varicose veins, sickle cell anemia, or cyanotic heart disease. Sickle cell trait is not considered to be a contraindication. The pill should probably be discontinued prior to elective surgery requiring prolonged bed rest.

Epilepsy

Seizure patients taking oral contraceptives should be observed closely for any increase in the number of seizures, associated with fluid retention. A middle- or low-dose pill should be selected, although several case reports have suggested that patients on anticonvulsant medications may metabolize contraceptive steroids more rapidly and therefore may be at greater risk from pill failure [16, 17].

Oligomenorrhea or amenorrhea

Scanty or absent withdrawal flow is most commonly associated with progestin-dominant pills (especially those containing norethindrone) and low-dose pills and may develop months or even several years after continuous usage. Reassurance may be all that is necessary, but most women feel more comfortable with a monthly period. Changing to an estrogen-dominant pill will usually lead to the resumption of menses.

After discontinuation of the pill, 2 percent of patients develop postpill amenorrhea [18]; approximately 95 percent of these revert to regular periods spontaneously or with clomiphene citrate within 12–18 months. Patients with a past history of oligomenorrhea or delayed menarche have an increased risk of post-pill amenorrhea; patients with a history of prolonged amenorrhea should strongly consider other forms of contraception.

Collagen disease

The pill is contraindicated in patients with lupus erythematosus (LE). Patients with rheumatoid arthritis may occasionally have increased symptoms. The pill has been reported to produce positive LE preparations and arthralgias in normal patients; these findings have disappeared when the pill has been discontinued [19, 20, 21, 22].

Diabetes

Pills with 50 μg or more of estrogen produce an abnormal glucose tolerance test in some patients. Patients with known diabetes mellitus may have increased insulin requirements. Chemical diabetics should probably use another form of contraception.

151

Jaundice

Because of occasional liver function abnormalities, patients with a past history of hepatitis should be given the pill only after liver function tests have remained normal for six months [23]. The pill is contraindicated in patients with cholestatic jaundice of pregnancy. An association between the pill and admissions to the hospital for gall-bladder surgery has been reported by the Boston Collaborative Drug Surveillance Program [14].

Changes in laboratory values

Miale and colleagues [24] have compiled a list of 100 laboratory tests that are potentially altered by oral contraceptives. Among the important effects noted are:

1. An increase in thyroxin (T_4) and a decrease in resin triiodothyronine (resin T_3), secondary to an increased thyroid-binding globulin. There is no change in free T_4 or the clinical status of the patient.
2. Slightly increased coagulation factors II, VIII, IX, X, and XII; factor VII is moderately increased. Compensatory mechanisms, including decreased serum antiplasmins and decreased clot tensile strength, are evident in many patients after two years of oral contraceptive use [25].
3. Increased triglycerides, cholesterol, and phospholipids [26]. The clinical risk has not been established, but another form of contraception should be used in patients with hyperlipidemia. A recent article reported two patients with type IV hyperlipidemia who developed pancreatitis on the pill [27].
4. Decreased serum folate. Long-term use of the pill may be associated with megaloblastic anemia.
5. Slightly increased sedimentation rate. Patients taking Oracon* have been shown to have sedimentation rates of 19–23 mm/hour compared to 10–15 mm/hour in controls [28].

Eye problems

Patients rarely may develop dry eyes from lack of tearing or corneal edema, which is probably an estrogenic effect. Contact lens users should be warned of possible problems. A progestin-dominant combination pill or the mini-pill may be better tolerated.

Depression

The increased incidence of depression among pill users appears to be related to an estrogen-induced change in tryptophan metabolism and

* A sequential pill that has been withdrawn from the market.

reduced cerebrospinal fluid serotonin levels. Supplementation with vitamin B_6 (30 mg/day) appears to lessen depression, but the long-term effects of giving high doses of this vitamin are unknown [29, 30]. Changing to a low-dose pill or the mini-pill may improve a patient's mood and libido.

Alopecia

Hair loss may be secondary to many stresses; therefore, it is difficult to establish the pill as a definite etiology in most cases. In rare instances, the pill may be a precipitating cause.

Cancer

Thus far there is no evidence of increased breast or cervical carcinoma associated with the use of oral contraceptives [31]. The pill may actually be protective against benign breast lesions after two years of continuous use [32, 33]. However, recent case reports have suggested a possible association between sequential pills (now withdrawn from the market) and endometrial cancer [34]. In addition, an association between benign hepatomas and the pill has been reported, with perhaps a higher risk for pills containing mestranol than those containing ethinyl estradiol [35, 36].

PATIENT EVALUATION WHEN PRESCRIBING ORAL CONTRACEPTIVES

The long list of side effects, indications, and contraindications makes it mandatory that the physician take a complete medical history and perform a general physical examination including blood pressure and breast and pelvic exams before prescribing the pill. Appropriate laboratory studies include urinalysis, hemoglobin, and Papanicolaou smear. A cholesterol and triglyceride test should be done on patients with a strong family history of arteriosclerotic heart disease or strokes. A blood test for syphilis once a year and a cervical culture for gonorrhea every six months is probably good screening in the sexually active teenage population.

For the patient with a history of regular periods and no particular indication for an estrogen- or progestin-dominant pill, selection of a medium-dose pill is appropriate (e.g., Ortho-Novum 1/50, Norinyl 1/50, Demulen, Ovral). Although a low-dose pill might seem preferable, the high incidence of breakthrough bleeding is unacceptable to many teenagers whose motivation for reliable contraception may be borderline. In well-motivated patients, a low-dose pill may be tried initially. Patients are instructed in the possible side effects—headaches, nausea, blood clots, and breakthrough bleeding—and given a three-month supply. Most pills are available in 21- and 28-day packages; the latter have seven placebo tablets. Most teenagers find it easier to remember to take a pill every day rather than 21 days on and 7 days off. If a pill is missed, the patient is instructed to take it as soon as she remembers; if two pills are missed, she is advised to take both pills and use an additional method of contraception (e.g., foam and condom, diaphragm, abstinence) for the remainder of the cycle. Written instructions often save phone calls (see Appendix 2). A teen-ager's fear and questions about the pill need to be carefully considered and answered; if a friend tells her after she leaves the physician's office that the pill "messes up the body" or "makes one sterile," she is apt to discontinue the medication in midcycle.

The follow-up visit at three months includes a blood pressure check and questioning about possible side effects. Not infrequently nausea and breakthrough bleeding that the patient experienced with the first package have disappeared with the third package. Adjustments in pill dosage can be made as suggested in the section on side effects. The patient is then seen at least every six months for renewal of the pill prescription, blood pressure and weight check, and breast and pelvic examination.

THE MINI-PILL

For the patient who seems unable to tolerate any estrogen dosage, the mini-pill (progestin only) may offer another option. The pregnancy rate is considerably higher (1.5–3.0 pregnancies/100 woman-years of use [up to 8/100 if pills are missed]) and may be unacceptable in some patients. The greatest disadvantage is the irregular bleeding that many patients experience. The pill is taken every day at the same time, not cyclically as are the combination pills. It has several modes of action: Foremost it alters cervical mucus, inhibiting sperm penetration; it also alters the endometrium in most women and in some patients blocks hypothalamic feedback mechanisms to eliminate the midcycle luteinizing hormone (LH) surge (and ovulation).

The thrombophlebitis risk has not been established but appears to be minimal. The coagulation changes associated with the combination pills are not evident with the progestins in short-term studies. Hypertension appears not to be a problem. Carbohydrate and lipid metabolism are probably not affected.

INTRAUTERINE DEVICES

Currently, approximately three million women in the United States are using intrauterine devices (IUDs) for contraception. The availability of the copper (Cu 7) and, soon, progesterone IUDs* for use in

---

* Progestasert (Alza) has been recently approved by the FDA. The incidence of bleeding, expulsion, infection, and pregnancy seems to be similar to the Cu 7; however, insertion may cause more pain, and the device must be removed and replaced every twelve months [37].

nulliparous women has increased the popularity of this method among adolescents. The Lippes Loop and Saf-T-Coil are still popular for postpartum women. The exact mechanism of action of IUDs is unknown. The inert IUDs (Lippes Loop, Saf-T-Coil) may prevent implantation by causing a low-grade endometritis; the contraceptive action of the Cu 7 is probably secondary to the effect of the copper on various endometrial enzymes [38].

The IUD should be inserted by a skilled physician. Insertion during the patient's period is simpler and ensures a nonpregnant uterus. Although nulliparous women previously experienced moderate cramps and occasional severe vagal reactions (syncope, seizures, bradycardia) with the insertion of the inert IUDs, the new small Cu 7 is associated with fewer complications. The patient should be informed about the side effects and complications of the Cu 7 before insertion [39–42].

Side Effects and Complications

Irregular bleeding and cramps

Cramps and bleeding are especially common in the first month of insertion but may persist. Monthly menstrual cramps may require stronger analgesics than previously. Approximately 7–13 percent of patients request removal of the IUD because of bleeding and pain.

Expulsion

Expulsion rates vary from 7–17 percent in the first two years after insertion, depending in part on the skill of the physician and the size of the uterus. Expulsion is most common in the first month after insertion. If an IUD is reinserted in a patient who has already expelled a device, the risk of second expulsion is considerably higher.

Infection

The rate of infection at the time of insertion is less than 1 percent; however, the reported incidence of pelvic inflammatory disease (PID) varies from 0.2–3.0/100 woman-years of use, depending on the patient population. The increased risk of PID may be caused in part by decreased use of the condom. Some cases of mild PID can be treated with the IUD in situ; however, in cases where the infection fails to come under prompt control within 48 hours, the device should be removed. Because of the risk of stirring up quiescent disease, the IUD is contraindicated in patients with a past history of recurrent PID or in patients with an acute pelvic infection within six months. If an IUD is inserted in a patient who had acute PID more than six months previously, ampicillin or tetracycline, 500 mg four times a day given two days before and seven days after insertion, may prevent a recurrence of the PID.

Many patients experience increased vaginal discharge with the IUD, probably secondary to irritation from the strings passing through the endocervical canal.

Pregnancy

Pregnancy rates with the Cu 7 vary from 1.1–2.5 pregnancies/100 woman-years of use. If a pregnancy occurs with the device in situ, the IUD should be removed because of the risk of infection and/or miscarriage in a midterm fetus. Removal may precipitate an abortion, but in general this is more acceptable early in a pregnancy and carries less risk to the woman.

The number of ectopic pregnancies is increased with the device in place; however, the seeming increase is probably related to the reduction in intrauterine pregnancies.

Perforation

The risk of perforation is probably less than 1/2000 insertions and depends on the size and position of the uterus and the experience of the physician. Because the Cu 7, unlike the inert Lippes Loop, stimulates a local inflammatory reaction, this device must be removed from the peritoneal cavity in cases of uterine perforation.

Except in cases of questionable follow-up or compliance with contraception, IUDs should be inserted four to eight weeks after delivery or therapeutic abortion to avoid the higher rates of expulsion and perforation.

Mortality

The mortality risk with the IUD is approximately 2/100,000 insertions.

PATIENT EVALUATION WITH THE IUD

After insertion of the IUD, the patient is shown how to check for the strings and is instructed to check once a week for one month and then after each period. Codeine, 30 mg every four hours, will alleviate cramps on the day of insertion. The patient is seen for a return visit at six weeks and then every six months to one year. The Cu 7 must be removed and replaced after 24 months because of decreased copper content; the Lippes Loop and Saf-T-Coil can probably remain in situ indefinitely.

The advantage of the IUD is that, once the device is in place, the patient does not have to remember to take one pill a day. After an abortion, some teenagers may find it easier to deal with their ambivalence about a repeat pregnancy with an IUD in place. In addition, the IUD is useful in adolescents with lupus erythematosus, sickle cell disease, renal disease, hypertension, and other chronic conditions that are contraindications to the use of the pill.

It is not unusual for an adolescent girl to express great concern about her body and its integrity and to be quite reluctant to accept a "piece of plastic" inside her. Often a friend who had heavy periods and cramps with an IUD will dissuade a patient from even considering the device. The physician must listen to the patient's concerns and answer each question with facts and diagrams of the uterus and vagina. The teenager must participate in the decision on what form of contraception is best for her.

DIAPHRAGM

Some adolescents are able to effectively use the diaphragm, a mechanical device fitted by the physician. In general, only an extremely motivated, mature adolescent who feels comfortable with her own body should rely on this form of contraception. The patient needs careful instructions, preferably written, on the use and care of the diaphragm; she should be shown how to feel for her cervix. A return appointment two to three weeks later to check for proper fit of the prescribed size allows the physician a chance to assess the patient's understanding and acceptance of this form of contraception. The obvious advantage of this method is the lack of side effects; however, the obvious disadvantage is the higher pregnancy rate.

The patient is given the following instructions:

1. Place one tablespoon of contraceptive jelly in the cup of the diaphragm and insert the diaphragm no more than two hours prior to intercourse. If the diaphragm is already in place and more than two hours have elapsed, insert an extra applicatorful of jelly into the vagina in front of the diaphragm. (Many women routinely insert the diaphragm every night.)
2. After inserting the diaphragm, check for the position of the cervix to make sure it is covered by the diaphragm.
3. Leave the diaphragm in place at least six hours after intercourse.
4. After removal, wash the diaphragm with mild soap (and dust it with cornstarch, if desired).
5. Once a week, hold the diaphragm up to a light and check for holes.
6. With any weight change of 10 pounds, consult your physician for a refitting.

FOAM AND CONDOM

The advantage of this form of contraception is that a knowledgeable teenager does not need a prescription to buy contraceptive foam or condoms; in addition the condom is the only form of birth control that lessens the risk of venereal disease. The disadvantage is the higher risk of pregnancy and the issue of motivation. Not infrequently, young men are unwilling to take responsibility for birth control, and a young woman may feel reluctant to force the contraception issue. In general, this form of contraception is best for the woman who has only occasional sexual relations.

Our instructions to the teenage girl are:

1. Insert the contraceptive foam into the vagina one hour or less *prior* to intercourse (not after intercourse).
2. Do not douche for at least six hours after intercourse.
3. Keep an extra condom with the contraceptive foam to lessen the risk of failure.

Specific names of foams (Emko, Delfen) should be mentioned, and a demonstration of how to fill the applicator is often given. Individual one-dose applicators (Conceptrol) are convenient but also more expensive than the refillable applicators.

DEPO-PROVERA

Medroxyprogesterone acetate (Depo-Provera) is an injectable contraceptive that has limited FDA approval. This drug has been used widely in developing countries but has been restricted here because of the rare occurrence of prolonged amenorrhea and sterility. It may be useful in certain retarded teenagers and in patients who have had repeated failure with other modes of contraception.

Depo-Provera, 150 mg intramuscularly every three months, suppresses the hypothalamic-ovarian axis and prevents the midcycle LH surge. In addition, it produces thinning and sometimes profound atrophy of the endometrium and increases the viscosity of the cervical mucus. The pregnancy rate is 0–0.3/100 woman-years.

The most important side effect is menstrual irregularities; patients often experience irregular spotting and occasionally very heavy periods in the first few months of therapy. The heavy bleeding usually responds to estrogen therapy so that a dilation and curettage is rarely indicated. After six months (or three injections of Depo-Provera), most patients are amenorrheic. If desired, withdrawal periods can be produced by administering 0.04 mg of ethinyl estradiol for seven to ten days each month. Other possible side effects of Depo-Provera include headaches, nervousness, weight gain, nausea, vomiting, decreased glucose tolerance, and possibly breast nodules. The risk of thromboembolic disease is probably not increased. Because of the possible risk of delay in the return of ovulatory cycles, the drug should not be used for spacing children. Data indicate, however, that 82 percent of 135 women became pregnant within 14 months of discontinuing Depo-Provera. This statistic can be compared with an 88 percent pregnancy rate twelve months after removal of an IUD and a 94 percent pregnancy rate twelve months after discontinuation of the pill [43].

THE "MORNING-AFTER" PILL

High-dose estrogens have been shown to lower the pregnancy risk significantly following unprotected intercourse. This form of therapy should in general be reserved for cases of rape and first intercourse. The only form of therapy approved by the FDA is diethylstilbestrol (DES); however, because of the risk of adenosis and adenocarcinoma of the vagina in offspring (see Chap. 10), it is imperative to (1) perform a pregnancy test and (2) inform the patient that, if she is already pregnant by a previous exposure, she should be willing to have an abortion. The patient should participate in the decision to use this drug. Other forms of estrogen therapy are now being substituted as documentation of their efficacy is reported. The medication should be given preferably within 24 hours and not later than 72 hours after unprotected intercourse and continued for five days. The doses are diethylstilbestrol, 25 mg twice a day for five days; *or* conjugated estrogens (Premarin), 25 mg twice a day for five days; *or* ethinyl estradiol (Estinyl), 2 mg twice a day for five days.

Enteric-coated DES is tolerated better than plain DES. All of the high-dose estrogens are associated with nausea and vomiting. Prochlorperazine (Compazine), 5–10 mg orally two hours prior to each dosage of estrogen, lessens the nausea. Other possible side effects include fluid retention (sometimes severe in patients with marked premenstrual edema), headaches, dizziness, menstrual irregularities, and breast soreness. The patient is warned against having intercourse for the remainder of the cycle. The failure rate is 0.03–0.3 percent [44, 45].

Insertion of a copper 7 IUD (Cu 7) is a reasonable alternative to estrogen therapy in the patient who needs "morning-after" protection for the first sexual experience and knows that she will continue to need contraception in the future.

REFERENCES

GENERAL REVIEWS OF BIRTH CONTROL

1. Kistner, R.W. (Ed.). *Reproductive Endocrinology.* New York: Medicine, Inc., 1973.
2. Kistner, R.W. The pill and IUD: Not perfect, but still the best we have. *Mod. Med.,* November 11, 1974. P. 36.
3. Cooke, C. Contraceptive usage among teenagers. *J. Am. Med. Wom. Assoc.* 28:639, 1973.
4. Topical and systemic contraceptive agents. *Med. Lett. Drugs Ther.* 16:37, 1974.

ORAL CONTRACEPTIVES

5. Garcia, G. R. The oral contraceptive: An appraisal and review. *Am. J. Med. Sci.* 253:718, 1967.
6. Nelson, J. H. Selecting the optimum oral contraceptive. *J. Reprod. Med.* 11:135, 1973.
7. Oral contraceptives and health. *Lancet* 1:1147, 1974.

8. Greenblatt, D. Oral contraceptives and hypertension. *Obstet. Gynecol.* 44:412, 1974.

9. Russell, R. P., et al. The pill and hypertension. *Johns Hopkins Med. J.* 127:287, 1970.

10. Crane, M.G., et al. Hypertension: Oral contraceptive agents and conjugated estrogens. *Ann. Intern. Med.* 74:13, 1971.

11. Weinberger, A. M. Oral contraceptives and hypertension. *Hosp. Practice* 10(5):65, 1975.

12. Tapia, H. R., et al. Effect of oral contraceptive therapy on renin-angiotensin system in normotensive and hypertensive women. *Obstet. Gynecol.* 41:643, 1973.

13. Inman, W., et al. Thromboembolic disease and the steroidal content of oral contraceptive pills: A report to the committee on safety of drugs. *Br. Med. J.* 2:203, 1970.

14. Boston Collaborative Drug Surveillance Program. Oral contraceptives and venous thromboembolic disease: Surgically confirmed gallbladder disease and breast tumours. *Lancet* 1:1399, 1973.

15. Collaborative Group in the Study of Stroke in Young Women. Oral contraception and increased risk of cerebral ischemia or thrombosis. *N. Engl. J. Med.* 288:871, 1973.

16. Janz, D., and Schmidt, D. Anti-epileptic drugs and failure of oral contraceptives. *Lancet* 1:1113, 1974.

17. Laengner, H., and Detering, K. Anti-epileptic drugs and failure of oral contraceptive drugs. *Lancet* 2:600, 1974.

18. Evrard, J., et al. Amenorrhea following oral contraception. *Am. J. Obstet. Gynecol.* 124:88, 1976.

19. Chapel, T., and Burns, R. Oral contraceptives and exacerbation of lupus erythematosus. *Am. J. Obstet. Gynecol.* 110:366, 1971.

20. Schleicher, E. LE cells after oral contraceptives. *Lancet* 1:821, 1968.

21. Bole, G., et al. Rheumatic symptoms and serological abnormalities induced by oral contraceptives. *Lancet* 1:323, 1969.

22. Kay, D. R., et al. Antinuclear antibodies, rheumatoid factor and C-reactive protein in serum in normal women using oral contraceptives. *Arthritis Rheum.* 14:239, 1971.

23. Adlercreutz, H., and Tenhunen, C. Some aspects of the interaction between natural and synthetic female sex hormones and the liver. *Am. J. Med.* 49:630, 1970.

24. Miale, J. B., et al. The effects of oral contraceptives on the results of laboratory tests. *Am. J. Obstet. Gynecol.* 120:264, 1974.

25. Mink, I., et al. Progestational agents and blood coagulation. *Am. J. Obstet. Gynecol.* 119:401, 1974.

26. Sachs, B., and Wolfman, L. Plasma lipid and lipoprotein changes during "pill-a-month" contraceptive steroid administration. *Am. J. Obstet. Gynecol.* 109:155, 1971.

27. Davidoff, F., et al. Hyperlipidemia and pancreatitis associated with oral contraceptive therapy. *N. Engl. J. Med.* 289:552, 1973.

28. Lorrain, J., et al. Effects of certain contraceptive hormones on blood coagulation. *Fertil. Steril.* 23:422, 1972.

29. Grant, E. C., et al. Effect of oral contraceptives on depressive mood changes. *Br. Med. J.* 3:777, 1968.

30. Larsson-Cohn, U. Oral contraceptives and vitamins: A review. *Am. J. Obstet. Gynecol.* 121:84, 1975.

31. Thomas, D. B. Relationship of oral contraceptives to cervical carcinogenesis. *Obstet. Gynecol.* 40:508, 1972.

32. Sartwell, P., et al. Epidemiology of benign breast lesions. *N. Engl. J. Med.* 288:551, 1973.
33. Vessey, M. P., et al. Oral contraceptives and breast neoplasia: A retrospective study. *Br. Med. J.* 3:719, 1972.
34. Kelley, H., et al. Adenocarcinoma of the endometrium in women taking oral contraceptives. *Obstet. Gynecol.* 47:200, 1976.
35. Baum, J., et al. Possible association between benign hepatomas and oral contraceptives. *Lancet* 2:926, 1973.
36. Edmondson, H., et al. Liver-cell adenomas associated with the use of oral contraceptives. *N. Engl. J. Med.* 294:470, 1976.

IUD
37. Progestasert—a new intrauterine contraceptive device. *Med. Lett. Drugs Ther.* 18:65, 1976.
38. Oster, G., and Salgo, M. The copper intrauterine device and its mode of action. *N. Engl. J. Med.* 293:432, 1975.
39. Levin, H., et al. The Cu 7: A metallic copper intrauterine device. *J. Reprod. Med.* 12:166, 1974.
40. Gibor, Y., et al. A prognostic indicator for the successful use of the Copper 7 intrauterine device. *J. Reprod. Med.* 11:205, 1973.
41. Lesenski, J., et al. Consideration of the relationship between the compliance of some intrauterine contraceptive devices and the expulsion rate. *J. Reprod. Med.* 11:205, 1973.
42. Orlans, F. Population Report Series B, Number 1. *Intrauterine Devices.* December, 1973.

DEPO-PROVERA
43. Rosenfield, A. G. Injectable long-acting progestogen contraception: A neglected modality. *Am. J. Obstet. Gynecol.* 120:537, 1974.

POSTCOITAL CONTRACEPTION
44. *FDA Drug Bulletin.* Post-coital diethylstilbestrol. May, 1973.
45. Morris, J. M., et al. Interception: The use of post-ovulatory estrogens to prevent implantation. *Am. J. Obstet. Gynecol.* 115:101, 1973.

15. Teenage Pregnancy

Unless the physician excludes all pubescent girls from his practice, he is going to be confronted with the diagnosis and management of unplanned pregnancies. The adolescent is faced with demands for premature heterosexual relationships in which intercourse is often defined as the major expression of "love." Failure to use reliable contraceptives has resulted in a rising birth rate among teenagers at a time when this rate has leveled off in the country as a whole.

FACTORS IN TEENAGE PREGNANCY

Why do teenagers become pregnant? Probably the most common statement we hear is, "I didn't think it would happen to me," which is somehow saying, "I'm special"; "I'm not really a woman." Although some teenagers may be ignorant of contraceptive devices, the majority are aware of contraception but fail to use the measures because of that "special" feeling. Some feel reluctant to destroy the spontaneity of the act by planning ahead. Since many teenagers are afraid to ask their physicians for birth control, the issue will never arise unless the patient has a trusting relationship with her doctor and is seen alone. Society has traditionally left contraception to the woman, but young men should be encouraged by the physician to accept responsibility for the prevention of unwanted pregnancies.

Although the majority of pregnant teenagers are neither emotionally disturbed nor promiscuous, emotional issues that may have precipitated the pregnancy should be carefully identified to prevent repetition. The loss of a parent by death or divorce often precedes a pregnancy. The pregnancy is viewed by the teenager as replacing that loss; the baby may be perceived as a doll-like person who will love and care for the teenager. Other teenagers may believe that the baby will help establish a lasting relationship with a boyfriend. The teenager who is threatened with punishment if she dares to become pregnant may feel compelled to rebel and test her mother's love. An occasional teenager will state with anger, "Well, I asked my mother for the pill and she refused, so this (pregnancy) is her fault." Pregnancy is often a plea for caring, and yet at the same time it may represent an announcement by the adolescent that she has become an adult. Unless these issues are resolved by counseling or psychotherapy, involving the family if possible, another pregnancy is likely to follow the abortion or delivery.

Confirmation of pregnancy depends to a large extent on suspicion. Some teenagers request appointments with the hope that the physician will accidentally discover the pregnancy. Often the presenting complaint is minor—a stomachache, constipation, or headaches—and the patient later admits to having missed her period only with direct questioning. Other adolescents may not have thought of the possibility and present with dizziness, syncope, nausea, or urinary frequency. The 2-minute urine pregnancy tests are easy screening tests (see Chap. 1).

COUNSELING THE PREGNANT ADOLESCENT

Counseling the pregnant teenager (and her family) is essential to alleviate the patient's anxiety and guilt and to reduce the long-term emotional sequelae. Active participation of the teenager in the decision-making is essential. Unfortunately, there is no "good" alternative to an unwanted pregnancy. With both adoption and abortion, the teenager must ultimately work through the guilt and loss. The teenager who elects to keep her baby may be emotionally unprepared to cope with the demands of child care.

When counseling pregnant teenagers, the physician will sense immediate differences between the 11–14-year-old and the 17–18-year-old girl. The younger girl tends to have many sexual fantasies and to deny the pregnancy until quite late; it is not unusual to see a 12-year-old girl twenty or even twenty-six weeks pregnant. The young adolescent is unable to take responsibility for her actions or even to connect pregnancy and motherhood. Since her decisions about what to do with the pregnancy may be related to angry feelings toward her parents that day, several visits may be necessary before a referral for abortion or obstetrical care is made. The 17- or 18-year-old girl is usually able to weigh more of the consequences of her action and to consider the choices available. The patient's needs, strengths, and defenses need to be assessed while formulating a plan [1, 2, 3]. A pregnancy information sheet such as that used at the Beth Israel Hospital in Boston is shown in Appendix 3.

The teenager not only has the final word on what decisions are to be made, but she must live with the decisions over her lifetime. Ambivalence about an unwanted pregnancy is a normal feeling and must be resolved as much as possible. Many teenagers fear sterility and other complications from abortion, which is perhaps related to guilt or the need for punishment. In order to work through the various options, the physician must be familiar with the surgical procedures and risks involved in abortion. In order to be fair to the teenager, the physician should be relatively unbiased ethically about abortion; if he/she is antiabortion, then the patient should be referred to a pregnancy counseling service. Admittedly it may be difficult to be unbiased about the prospect of the young adolescent keeping her baby because of the frequent problems seen with teenage marriages and out-of-wedlock babies.

Not infrequently the teenager finds it easier to have the physician tell her mother the diagnosis. Parents may feel very guilty or very angry. Unfortunately, if a mother expresses her demands for abortion or continuing the pregnancy too emphatically, she may push her daughter in the opposite direction. Since the teenager generally will continue to live with her parents, a solution acceptable to both parents and teenager needs to be evolved through counseling. Introducing the topic of birth control after the pregnancy is essential, for many teenagers and parents feel that "it won't happen again." The likelihood of repetition should be emphasized.

ABORTION

For the teenager who desires a therapeutic abortion, a quick pelvic examination and recording of the last menstrual period (LMP) will help with the appropriate referral. It should be remembered that pregnancies are dated from the LMP even though ovulation usually occurs at least two weeks later. By rectal or vaginal examination, the eight-week uterus feels about the size of an orange; the twelve-week uterus is approximately the size of a grapefruit. If the pediatrician is unfamiliar with pelvic exams an abdominal exam is useful. The twelve-week uterus is just palpable at the symphysis pubis; the twenty-week uterus is at the level of the umbilicus; a sixteen-week uterus is midway in between (Fig. 15-1).

First-Trimester Abortion

Before twelve weeks of pregnancy, an abortion is performed by suction curettage. This can be done under general or local anesthesia in a hospital or free-standing abortion clinic. Most teenagers do well with general anesthesia given in an ambulatory setting; the patient arrives at eight o'clock in the morning (with nothing taken orally after midnight) and goes home around noontime. She is told that the abortion is like a "heavy period," and that she will continue to have her period for several days after the procedure. She is encouraged to start on birth control pills three days later. Complications depend on the skill of the gynecologist and the duration of the pregnancy—i.e., there are fewer problems with interrupting a pregnancy at eight weeks than at twelve weeks. Fever and abdominal pain occurring within one week of the abortion may signal infection; continued bleeding and abdominal cramps may indicate retained products of conception. In both situations the patient should be referred to the gynecologist who performed the procedure for appropriate therapy. Infection is usually treated with bed rest and antibiotics, either in or out of the hospital; subinvolution is treated with ergonovine (Ergotrate), 0.2 mg three times daily for three days, and possibly repeat curettage.

A review of 26,000 first-trimester ambulatory abortions in New

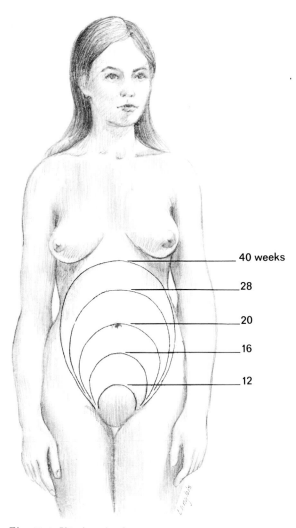

Fig. 15-1. Uterine size in pregnancy.

York City (July 1, 1970 to August 1, 1971) showed the following complications [4]:

1. Uterine perforation (1.4/1,000): approximately one-third required laparotomy.
2. Incomplete abortion with repeat curettage necessary (3.5/1,000).
3. Infections (15/1,000).
4. Hemorrhage (2.1/1,000).
5. No deaths.

Although follow-up was not complete, these statistics are similar to those reported from other clinics [5]. Patients with chronic diseases, including heart disease, renal disease, and sickle cell anemia, were excluded because of the ambulatory setting of this type of clinic. Although this has not been substantiated in recent studies, repeated first-trimester abortions may be associated with an increased incidence of cervical incompetence and prematurity during a normal pregnancy.

SECOND-TRIMESTER ABORTION

Only a few exceptionally skilled obstetricians are willing to undertake a suction curettage of a 13- or 14-week uterus. In general, most patients beyond 12 weeks need a saline- or prostaglandin-induced abortion performed on an inpatient basis between 16 and 24 weeks of pregnancy. Under local anesthesia a catheter is inserted into the uterus, amniotic fluid is withdrawn, and an equal volume of saline or prostaglandins is injected. Within 12 to 36 hours, the patient goes into labor and delivers a dead fetus. Sedation is required and supportive counseling is essential. Contraindications to saline include chronic renal disease, cardiac disease, and severe anemia. The complication rate rises with the increasing size of the uterus; complications include infection, retained products of conception, coagulopathy, and rarely mortality [6]. The Mount Sinai Hospital in New York reported the following incidences of complications in a series of second-trimester abortions [7]:

1. Infection (23/1,000).
2. Retained placenta (129/1,000).
3. Hemorrhage (> 500 cc: 23/1,000).
4. Failure of induction (3/1,000).
5. Mortality (.1/1,000).

FOLLOW-UP COUNSELING

The physician should be familiar with the community's resources before a pregnant teenager appears, since the supportive counseling and the gynecological care at different hospitals and clinics are variable. Although a woman with three or four children may have few second thoughts about an abortion, the teenager needs time to participate in a decision about the pregnancy. Otherwise she will see herself essentially as a sexually active person who was stupid enough to get pregnant and certainly not fit to be a mother. Counseling before and after the procedure is essential and should support the patient's decision as the right one for her. The question, "Are you sure you want an abortion?" at the time of the procedure may undermine a carefully thought-out decision. Nurses, doctors, and aides who are antiabortion should not care for these patients because they may intensify guilt and anxiety in the young adolescent.

Follow-up visits two weeks postabortion and then at least every three months for a year will allow the patient a chance to verbalize her feelings. Ambivalence about the pregnancy and abortion may recur. A teenager may feel the need to discontinue her pills for several days when the ambivalent feelings emerge; thus the intrauterine device (IUD) may have a lower pregnancy rate among postabortion patients even though the theoretical pregnancy rate is higher. The abortion date itself often takes on a magical quality for the teenager, and she may return one year after the abortion with psychosomatic complaints and depression.

CONTINUING THE PREGNANCY TO TERM

The teenager who desires to continue her pregnancy to term should receive special prenatal care. An increased incidence of toxemia [8] and low-birth-weight babies has been noted among teenagers; low-birth-weight infants are probably the result of the poor nutrition in the mother. Younger teenagers tend to have more severe preeclampsia than older teenagers [9]. Currently, there are 200 special programs in this country for pregnant adolescents to help prepare them for delivery, motherhood, and future family planning. The adolescent is seen for frequent visits by a multidisciplinary team consisting of a doctor, nurse, dietician, and social worker. Informal discussion groups led by a nurse help to educate the adolescent in nutrition, basic physiology, types of anesthesia, fetal monitoring, breast versus bottle feeding, postpartum care, and contraceptives. In communities without such programs, a sympathetic nurse in the obstetrician's office may fill a similar educational role.

The number of repeat unplanned pregnancies depends to a large extent on the patient's rapport with her physician or special team and her knowledge of available contraception. Postpartum insertion of an IUD may seem preferable to the doctor, but the patient's wishes clearly need to be respected and alternatives discussed.

REFERENCES

1. Addelson, F.   Induced abortion: Source of guilt or growth. *Am. J. Orthopsychiatry* 43:815, 1973.
2. Nadelson, C.   Abortion counselling: Focus on adolescent pregnancy. *Pediatrics* 54:765, 1974.
3. Nadelson, C., et al.   The pregnant teenager. *Psychiatr. Opinion* 12:1, 1975.
4. Nathanson, B. N.   Ambulatory abortion: Experience with 26,000 cases. *N. Engl. J. Med.* 286:403, 1972.
5. Hodgson, J., and Portmann, K.   Complications of 10,453 consecutive first trimester abortions: A prospective study. *Am. J. Obstet. Gynecol.* 120:802, 1974.

6. Stim, E.   Saline abortion. *Obstet. Gynecol.* 40:247, 1972.
7. Kerenyi, T.   Unpublished data, 1974.
8. Duenhoelter, J., et al.   Pregnancy performance of patients under 15 years of age. *Obstet. Gynecol.* 46:49, 1975.
9. Zackler, J. (Ed.).   *The Teenage Pregnant Girl.* Springfield, Ill.: Thomas, 1975.

SELECTED READING

Marinoff, S., and Schonholz, D.   Adolescent pregnancy. *Pediatr. Clin. North Am.* 19(3):795, 1972.
Wallace, H. M.   A study of services and needs of teenage pregnant girls in large cities in the U.S. *Am. J. Public Health* 63:5, 1973.

16. Rape

Rape is an increasing problem, with psychosocial, medical, and legal implications. The majority of rapes are probably never reported to the police. Many young girls and teenagers may never even report the rape to family or physician and may, therefore, never receive appropriate care and counseling. Sometimes an unwanted pregnancy or neurotic symptoms may force a patient to reveal an event that she had attempted to deny.

What constitutes rape? By definition, rape is the introduction of the penis within the genitalia of the victim by force, fear, or fraud. Neither ejaculation nor laceration of the hymen is necessary for the allegation. Statutory rape is coitus with a female below the age of consent (in most states, age 16). Sexual molestation is noncoital sexual contact without consent.

In all cases, it is extremely important that the patient be given sympathetic medical care. The initial encounter with a medical clinic or emergency ward should be a positive experience. Of prime importance is the presence of a sympathetic female figure (ideally, an experienced nurse or counselor) who can guide the patient through the emergency ward procedures, the pelvic examination, and the legal systems (if desired). Otherwise the encounter, especially the pelvic exam, may seem to the patient to be a repeat of the rape.

PATIENT EVALUATION

In all cases of alleged rape or molestation, medical data should be carefully collected and recorded because of the legal implications. The history, written in the patient's words, should include such details as time, place, circumstances, others present, and resistance. The patient should be asked if she has bathed, douched, or urinated since the assault. Menstrual and contraception history should be included. The physician should not try to decide whether rape or seduction has occurred on the basis of the patient's emotional response to the trauma, for clearly some patients will be tearful, tense, and hysterical, and others will appear controlled or subdued.

After the history is obtained, the patient should be told of the need for a thorough physical examination to assess injuries and to collect laboratory specimens. Consent forms should be signed for all procedures and should be witnessed by a nurse or other individual in the emergency ward or clinic. The physical examination should include:

1. A description of the patient's general appearance, emotional state, and especially the condition of clothing (i.e., neat, disheveled, torn, having bloodstains).

2. A general physical examination, with a notation of hematomas, bruises, edema, abrasions, lacerations, and other evidences of struggle (e.g., hair or skin beneath the fingernails, scratches).
3. A pelvic examination, with careful inspection of the external genitalia, urethra, vagina, cervix, and anus. If possible, a vaginal examination should be done with a dry or water-moistened speculum (no lubricant) in order to preserve the findings. If the hymen is tight, samples may be obtained from the introitus with a saline-moistened Q-Tip or eyedropper.

LABORATORY TESTS

The necessary laboratory procedures include:

1. A swab from the vaginal pool and from any suspicious areas around the vulva. The swab(s) should be protected in a test tube and saved for the police. A police laboratory can test for acid phosphatase and the blood group antigens of semen and perform precipitin tests against human sperm and blood.
2. Two swabs from the vaginal pool. The slides should be marked with the patient's name and date and labeled #1 and #2. Slide #1 is streaked with one swab and placed in Papanicolaou's (Pap) fixative for H & E staining as a permanent record. On slide #2, one drop of saline is mixed with the second swab. A coverslip is applied, and the slide is examined under the high dry power of a microscope for red blood cells and motile sperm. The presence of motile sperm implies sexual contact within 28 hours; nonmotile sperm may persist in the vagina for up to 48 hours. If the smear is positive, it should be placed in the Pap fixative. The absence of sperm does not imply that the fluid is not seminal, for ejaculates may contain no sperm in patients who have had a vasectomy or who have primary azoospermia [1].
3. Endocervical and rectal cultures for gonorrhea.
4. Serology for syphilis.
5. Pregnancy test to detect preexisting pregnancy (especially if menses are late or irregular).
6. Complete blood count (CBC).

All laboratory specimens for the pathology laboratory or police should be delivered personally by the doctor or nurse involved in the case, and properly signed receipts should be obtained.

TREATMENT

Prophylactic treatment to abort syphilis, gonorrhea, and possible pregnancy should be discussed with the patient. If she agrees, she should be treated with:

1. Procaine penicillin G, 4.8 million units intramuscularly, and probenecid, 1 gm orally just before the injection (for alternative therapy see page 114). A follow-up serology for syphilis is necessary if
   alternative therapy is used.
2. Diethylstilbestrol or conjugated estrogen (Premarin) to prevent
   pregnancy (see page 158 for indications and informed consent).

A follow-up appointment is given for one week later. A repeat pelvic
examination should be done only if necessary to assess healing of
injuries. A repeat serology for syphilis, pregnancy test, and cervical
culture (if it can be obtained atraumatically) are done at the six-week
follow-up visit. Clearly the above procedure should be modified when
a patient presents days or weeks after an assault.

AFTERMATH: IMPORTANCE OF COUNSELING

In general, responsibility for reporting the incident belongs to the
patient and her parents (if the patient is less than 18 years old).
Although improvements are in sight, prosecution may intensify the
guilt and shame of the victim. Questions such as "What were you doing out late?" or "What did you expect?" or "Why didn't you struggle?" may force the patient to feel that she was somehow responsible for the rape. On the other hand, unless rapes are reported and
prosecuted, the prevention of further violence is jeopardized.

Assessment of the teenager and her family is vital. In situations
where another family member is involved in the rape or molestation,
psychosocial intervention is usually necessary for the whole family.
For example, if a mother unconsciously "sets up" her daughter to be
raped by the father or stepfather, the approach should be similar to
that now available for battered children.

The availability of counseling should be stressed to the teenager.
Even if she seems nonverbal or appears to be coping well, the counselor can often play an educational and supportive role in the initial
interviews. The patient needs reassurance about her intactness and
her femininity. She may need the opportunity to tell and retell her
story to a caring, sympathetic person. Ideally, an experienced counselor should be available at the time the rape is reported and should be
willing to follow up the patient by telephone or home visits. It is not
unusual for a patient to have somatic reactions in the first several
weeks following a rape—muscle soreness, headaches, fatigue, stomach
pains, dysuria, sleep disturbances, and nightmares. Most rape victims
express an extreme fear of physical violence and death. Many older
women move and change their telephone numbers [2].

In the course of counseling, it is important to acknowledge to the
patient that she may feel increasingly vulnerable and helpless and
that the rape incident may interfere with her ability to form trusting

relationships, especially with men. It is not unusual for women to experience extreme shame, guilt, and loss of self-esteem after a rape, insisting that they might have somehow avoided the incident. The response of parents, doctors, and friends often fosters this guilt in the victim and forces her to regard the rape as a sexual act rather than the violent crime she perceived. Parents and boyfriends may respond by being overprotective at a time when the teenager is striving for independence; her sense of adequacy is thus further questioned. The young adolescent is often reluctant to return to school because of the fear that peer groups "will whisper behind her back." Stating this as a problem and suggesting that some of this behavior may be related to the feeling, "I'm glad it did not happen to me, but I wonder what it was like," may relieve the patient of some of her anxiety. Preventive measures, such as avoiding walking alone or hitchhiking, can be emphasized without making the patient feel that she shares the blame for the incident.

It is difficult to predict the long-term sequelae of a rape because victims cope with stress in many different ways. However, it is clear that later sexual disturbances are common when the first sexual experience occurs in the context of violence and degradation. The other issues that tend to emerge later include (1) mistrust of men, (2) phobic reactions, and (3) neurotic symptoms of anxiety and depression precipitated by events that remind the victim of the original episode [3].

Despite the need to work through these issues both at the time of crisis and in later years, the teenager often expresses reluctance to continue follow-up care because repeated encounters with the hospital setting remind her of the original incident. Thus, the initial counseling interviews should assess the patient's strengths in coping with stress and emphasize the availability of follow-up or referral. Telephone contact should be continued if at all possible. Involving a friend or relative whom the patient views as supportive is often helpful. The emphasis must be on working through the long-term problems that confront the rape victim and not merely dealing with the crisis of days or weeks.

REFERENCES

1. Breen, T., et al. The molested young female: Evaluation and therapy of alleged rape. *Pediatr. Clin. North Am.* 19(3):717, 1972.
2. Burgess, A., and Holmstom, L. Rape trauma syndrome. *Am. J. Psychiatry* 131:981, 1974.
3. Notman, M., and Nadelson, C. The rape victim: Psychodynamic considerations. *Am. J. Psychiatry* 133:408, 1976.

17. Sex Education

Robert P. Masland, Jr., M.D.*

The term *sex education* calls forth a variety of responses from parents, children, adolescents, and young adults, usually in accord with early family experiences, level of formal education, and current lifestyle. Perhaps the most important aspect of sex education is the role played by the parents. Compatible parents, or indeed a single parent or a parent surrogate who is both thoughtful and considerate of the child's needs, usually have little difficulty dealing with the concerns of both parent and child in the area of sex information, attitudes, and values. Children appreciate the stability provided by strong, caring parents and respond in a positive fashion as they incorporate sexuality into their character and personality development. Since society seems to perplex all of us, with the constant being change rather than consistency, physicians in family practice, pediatrics, and adolescent medicine must be available to provide assistance for parents and children in sex education. What was acceptable to society yesterday no longer applies today. The resulting confusion can and does lead to breakdown in communication in the best family situations. Physicians must be willing to provide both care and information for their young patients in an atmosphere of trust and confidentiality. Sex education is most effective for the adolescent when it involves a physician-patient relationship that is truly confidential. Parents can be counseled in a manner that recognizes their need for support, without betraying the confidence of the youngster.

When we speak of sex education, we always seem to imply that it is for the young, and in particular for the adolescent, and more particularly for the adolescent girl, since it is the adolescent girl who is most vulnerable for the obvious reason: When she is sexually active, she runs the risk of becoming pregnant. To be sure, we do worry a bit about the adolescent boy, but when sex information has been given to young boys, the emphasis has tended to be on the discussion of masturbation, wet dreams, and homosexuality. Rarely do boys have an opportunity to discuss feelings, physical and emotional, toward girls. Opportunity for such discussions in groups of boys only, and then in mixed boy-girl groups, has the capacity to make boys and girls think and act more responsibly both socially and sexually. We teach our toddlers and prepubertal children the joys of sharing and loving;

---

* Assistant Professor of Pediatrics, Harvard Medical School; and Chief, Division of Adolescent Medicine, The Children's Hospital Medical Center, Boston, Massachusetts.

then adolescence enters the picture and it is no longer permissible to share and love, at least not in any way that involves sexual feelings. It is my belief that sex education enhances the capacity of the individual adolescent to make sexual decisions that are both informed and thoughtful. When I say thoughtful, I mean thoughtful of the needs of the other individual with whom a sexual relationship has evolved. By "sexual relationship" I mean a relationship that has created a situation which may or may not include sexual intercourse.

ROLE OF PARENTS IN SEX EDUCATION

All too often parents are not active participants in formal sex education for their children. However, parents do provide models of behavior for the children in a passive sense. Affection, respect, and love between father and mother are unmistakable signals that are picked up by children of all ages. A man or woman raising a child or children without a partner for the child to observe is handicapped. Most single parents make a considerable effort to involve good people of the opposite sex in family activities in order to provide role models. It is expected that children will learn a great deal about how to behave as an adult by observing adult behavior. It is not uniformly true that a strong, caring marriage will lead to offspring who will develop similar relationships, but it does help! I am certain that we can recall children who have overcome impossible family conditions and have gone on to become adolescents and adults capable of considerate, responsible, and responsive sexual behavior; but it does seem to be less hazardous for a child who grows up in a supportive family atmosphere. Hence the role of the physician who cares for young patients is twofold: He is an advocate for the adolescent, a sustainer for the parents. In this way the physician may be able to maintain a family that is already supportive, and for those families in disarray, the physician may create a semblance of order as the advocate-sustainer. A home where information can be exchanged without rancor or fear of retribution is the preferred setting for dealing with the ultimate questions of young people: What does it mean to be a woman? What does it mean to be a man?

Adolescents require guidelines, a point of reference if you will, either to accept or rebel against. In the area of sexual behavior it is important for parents to answer questions with facts when known, and always with a statement, not a lecture, of personal opinion. Right or wrong, consistent or inconsistent, a parental opinion has to be expressed on sexual matters as a benchmark for children to recall. Children can and will obtain sexual information outside the home; more often than not this information is a mixture of truth, half-truth, lies, and myths. Such information must be reviewed with adults who have a rapport with the young person, and the preferred adults are the parents. The physician must be available as a backup for the parents, or to take over when the parents are lacking in information which the child must have in addition to parental feelings. There are many highly competent counselors available for young people in addition to parents and physicians: Teachers, psychologists, guidance counselors, clergy, and social workers are key people to whom adolescents may turn when perplexed by sexual issues. A counselor may not be able to state a personal opinion quite as easily as a parent. In fact, the counselor who talks too much and fails to listen and then responds in an objective manner may be ineffective with the adolescent. Adults are watched carefully by the adolescent, which underscores the well-known statement that adolescents are influenced as much, if not more, by adult action as by adult speeches.

Decisions must be made by the adolescent in all areas of life, but most particularly with regard to sexual interaction with members of the same and opposite sex. Points of view, which may be quite different, can be exchanged between adult and adolescent. In the home, with parent and child locked in emotional conflict, there may be little room for discussion of the highly charged matter of sexual activity. Parents are traditionally more comfortable in an extreme posture that defines clearly to the child an irrevocable position. The inflexible, "thou shalt not" parent is all too familiar. No discussion necessary; case dismissed! At the opposite pole we find the confused parents, unable to make decisions for themselves or for their children. In this case the result is a home filled with doubts, deceit, chaos, permissiveness, and irresponsibility. Parents of both types, inflexible and confused, can be equally inconsistent. Vacillation by adults on many issues can and does lead to exploitation by the adolescent. When the parent and adolescent are no longer able to communicate in a reasonable fashion, then it is appropriate to seek professional help. With proper support from a professional—and two counselors may be needed, one for the adolescent and one for the parent—one can hope to temper the inflexible parent's opinion and the adolescent's stubborn rebellion.

ROLE OF THE PHYSICIAN AS COUNSELOR

If the physician is to be the counselor, then the adolescent must be seen alone in the physician's office. Ample opportunity must be provided for the adolescent to state the problem, and the physician must be willing to listen without interruption. If the adolescent's story does not include information concerning sexual activity, then it is perfectly proper for the physician to ask these questions.

The adolescent's story may lead the physician in the direction of asking questions concerning a variety of sexual issues. For example, there may be considerable tension in the home relating to the parents' disapproval of the daughter's boyfriend. In her conversation with the physician, the daughter may not want to reveal her primary concern, which may be her questions concerning birth control. If sexual activity is suspected by the physician, then the question should be clearly stated so that the adolescent knows that specific information is required. The physician must stress, once again, the confidentiality of the doctor-patient relationship. The physician who listens, asks the appropriate questions, and provides medical information in a confidential manner will have little or no difficulty dealing with adolescents' sexuality problems. One cannot dictate the physician's life-style, but one can be certain that the manner in which this information is presented will reflect the physician's attitude. The physician may not be in agreement with the adolescent's life-style, but to be an effective counselor for adolescents, one must not act in a judgmental manner.

The question of masturbation may be an important issue for boys and girls, and again, I would urge that the physician listen to the young person before asking the direct questions that must be asked if one is to provide relief for the patient. The anxiety and guilt that some young patients experience with regard to masturbation cannot be overemphasized. Reassurance that masturbation is not harmful to the body can and will put the problem in proper perspective with the adolescent patient.

Homosexual feelings, and perhaps actions, often surface during early adolescence. It is perfectly normal for boys and girls to have close friends of the same sex, not only in early adolescence but throughout adolescence and adult life. When the friendship becomes a physical relationship, there may be some very real anxieties expressed by the adolescent boy or girl. If the physician is comfortable dealing with the subject of homosexuality, at least in the preliminary stage of evaluating whether or not the problem is a serious one for the patient, then the physician can and must ask the right questions and provide both answers and recommendations. However, it may be necessary for the physician to refer the patient for a psychiatric consultation. When a psychiatric consultation is requested, the patient must know that the reason for the referral is that a psychiatrist knows a great deal more than the physician about the subject of homosexuality and therefore is the ideal person to deal with the questions raised.

The increasing number of young adolescent girls who are taking the birth control pill has resulted in a new situation for adolescent society. Heretofore, the young boy had always been thought of as the aggressive one, but now we find adolescent girls on the pill equally aggressive in their desire for sexual activity. For some young boys this has created a problem, particularly in the area of sexual performance. The boy who is unsure of himself, and certainly there are many boys in this category, may turn away from heterosexual interests.

The boy who shies away from girls because he fears that he would be inadequate in a sexual encounter may find himself drifting into homosexual liaisons. It is a new situation for physicians to think of boys withdrawing from heterosexual activity, and it is well worth remembering when physicians see young male patients in their offices.

SEX EDUCATION IN THE COMMUNITY

Education in adolescent behavior, including sexuality, for parents and children can be achieved only with the approval and support of the adult community. The physician with interest and training in the developmental problems of children and youth must be the focal point in the community for information and instruction in adolescent behavior. Although elective courses in human sexuality are available in most medical schools, these courses are not given high priority in student education. As a consequence, only a small number of young physicians can be considered reasonably knowledgeable in the field of sexuality. It is not that the practicing physician lacks information regarding the physical aspects of sex but rather that physicians have not been sensitized to the specific emotional needs of young people and their parents when this information is dispensed. For the interested physician who wishes additional training in the area of sexuality, there are postgraduate courses, textbooks, and clinics devoted to this subject. A good beginning would be to contact SIECUS (Sex Information and Education Council of the United States*); through this organization the physician will receive a list of recommended reading material, both at the professional and the parent-patient level. Additional information may be obtained from the American Medical Association and from state and local medical societies.

When a community looks to the medical profession for guidance in developing a program for sex education, it is essential that two issues be met head on: the amount of information the adult community wishes to include in the program and the necessity of having young people on the committee that devises the curriculum. It is absolutely essential that the program include a thorough discussion of the biological growth and development of boys and girls during adolescence. The wide range of normal biological growth must be covered so that boys and girls at different stages of development will understand that the differences in size, shape, and configuration during early adolescence are to be expected and therefore can be understood as a normal part of growth and development. This concept may be a difficult one for the short boy or the tall girl, the early maturing boy or girl, and for the thin or fat adolescent. Parents must be aware of the wide

* SIECUS, 1855 Broadway, New York, N.Y. 10023.

range of normal development so that they may deal with the problems at home with sensitivity rather than ridicule and ignorance.

I am confident that most adults will have no quarrel with a program that includes information on venereal disease, but there will be conflict on the subjects of pregnancy, abortion, birth control, and psychosocial counseling. A bond of trust must be developed between the adult leaders, adolescents, and physicians concerned with the format and content of the course. The program that is best for the community will include an opportunity to discuss all of the important issues appropriate for the chronological and biological age level of the participants. Approval by both adult and adolescent groups will assure a favorable response from the community at large.

Small discussion groups (10–15 young people) are the preferred medium. Again, according to the decision of the adult-adolescent committee, the groups may be single sex or integrated. Grouping according to age would be best, although one must keep in mind that there is a wide range of biological growth from age 10 to 16 years. Regardless of how well the group has been set up, there will be young people of different levels of sexual awareness in every group, a fact which must be taken into account by the group leaders. Dealing with this disparity in the group must be discussed in the early sessions. Discussion groups, led by a person trained in group dynamics as well as human sexuality, have as a goal the resolution of conflict, misinformation, and fantasies regarding sexual behavior. It should not be the intent of the group to discuss only matters of sexual behavior; many other problems that concern adolescents can and should be brought up for group interaction. In addition to family living problems, one can anticipate that drugs, alcohol, and school disciplinary issues will be a part of the group discussion. There may be participants in each group who will require individual counseling; a skilled leader will detect these people and provide special and separate counseling for them.

It is not inappropriate to consider counseling services for preadolescent boys and girls. One hesitates to place an upper and lower age limit for availability of these services, but group discussions might begin as early as 9 or 10 years of age in a community where the parents accept the idea of making sex information available prior to puberty. Group meetings and individual sessions as required ought to be possible for all young people. One cannot begin too early to provide information for children in human sexuality.

SUGGESTED READING

1. Katchadourian, H. A., and Lunde, D. T. *Fundamentals of Human Sexuality*. New York: Holt, Rinehart, and Winston, 1972.
2. Leif, H. I.   Medical Aspects of Sexuality. In P. B. Beeson and W. Mc-

Dermott (Eds.), *Textbook of Medicine* (14th ed.). Philadelphia: Saunders, 1971. Pp. 581–585.
3. Sex Information and Education Council of the United States (SIECUS). *Sexuality and Man.* New York: Scribner, 1970.
4. Sorenson, R. C. *Adolescent Sexuality in Contemporary America.* New York: World, 1973.

Appendix 1. Excretion of 17-Ketosteroids

The measurement of urinary 17-ketosteroids includes mainly the excretion of androsterone and etiocholanolone. The main precursor is dehydroepiandrosterone (DHA), but metabolites of testosterone, androstenedione, and cortisol also contribute to this value. The excretion begins to rise between ages 6 and 8 as shown in Table 1 and in Figure 1.

Table 1. Values of 17-Ketosteroids (mg in 24 hours)

Age	Normal	Congenital Adrenal Hyperplasia
0–2 weeks	<0.5 (up to 2.5 mg)	1–5
2 weeks–6 months	<0.5	1–10
7–12 months	<0.5	3–10
1–5 years	<1	4–30
6–9 years	1–3	11–40
10–15 years	3–11	15–50
15 years	5–15	15–80

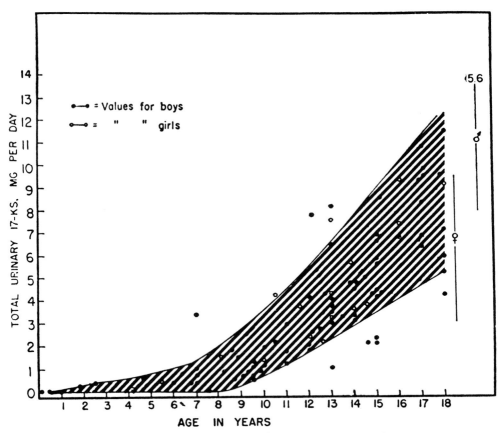

Fig. 1. *Urinary 17-ketosteroid excretion during childhood and adolescence.*
(Reprinted from N. Talbot et al.   Excretion of 17-ketosteroids by normal
and by abnormal children. Am. J. Dis. Child. 65 :354, 1943. Copyright, 1943,
American Medical Association, by permission.)

Appendix 2. Instruction Sheet for Taking 28-Day Contraceptive Pills (The Children's Hospital Medical Center, Boston)

1. The name of your birth control pill is _____.
2. If you are taking pills for the first time, take the first pill of your first package on the Sunday following the first day of your next period, even if you have stopped bleeding before that day. If your period begins on Sunday, start taking the pills on the same day.
3. Take one pill every day without fail. As soon as you finish your last pill in the package, the next day start the first pill in a new package. This means that you will be taking the pills even during the days you are having a period.
4. Always take the pill at approximately the same time each day. The best time is one-half hour after a good meal or snack, but whatever schedule you set up, you should stick to it.
5. *If you forget to take pills:*
   a. If you forget one pill, take the pill you forgot as soon as you remember; then take your regular pill for that day at the time you usually take your pill.
   b. If you forget two or more pills, take the pills you forgot as soon as you remember; then take your regular pill for the day at your regular time. A second method—foam, condom, or diaphragm—should be used during sexual relations until your period begins, but *continue* taking your pills.
6. Your period will appear normally sometime during your last week of pills in each package.
7. As long as you are taking the pills according to the directions above, you are completely protected against getting pregnant. Protection starts with the first pill.
8. *If you purchase your pills in three-month supplies, you must keep the pharmacy label from the first package and bring it with you when you go to the pharmacy to get refills. This label has your prescription number on it.*
9. If you have any problems or questions, please call us.

Appendix 3. Pregnancy Information Sheet (Beth Israel Hospital, Boston)

In order to provide more personalized medical care, we are asking you to fill out this form. If you need help, please ask the secretary. You do not have to answer any of the questions if you choose not to.

1. What made you first think you were pregnant?
2. When were you sure that you were pregnant?
3. What did you do then?
4. How did you feel when you were sure you were pregnant?
   Good ___ So-So ___ Sad ___ Angry ___
5. How do you feel now about being pregnant?
   Good ___ So-So ___ Sad ___ Angry ___
6. Who knows you're pregnant?
   family ___ husband ___ nobody ___ friends ___ boyfriend ___ other ___
7. Are they pleased?
   family ___ husband ___ nobody ___ friends ___ boyfriend ___ other ___
8. Are they displeased?
   family ___ husband ___ nobody ___ friends ___ boyfriend ___ other ___
9. If you are under 18, do you live with your family? Yes ___ No ___ Do you plan to stay there? Yes ___ No ___
10. If you are under 18, do you attend school? Yes ___ No ___ Would you like to continue? Yes ___ No ___
11. In the past six months, have there been any changes in your life (marriage, death of someone close, loss of job, etc.)?

If yes, explain.

12. Were you bothered by any of the following? (Check which ones)

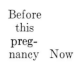

	Before this pregnancy	Now
Trouble sleeping	___	___
Poor appetite	___	___
Bad dreams	___	___
Trouble concentrating on job, school	___	___
Not enjoying doing things I usually like	___	___
Feel nervous	___	___
Feel sad	___	___
Feel irritable	___	___
Feel nauseated	___	___
Weight loss	___	___

13. What do you want to do about this pregnancy?
    Continue pregnancy ___
    Continue pregnancy and have baby adopted ___
    End pregnancy ___
    Don't know ___
14. Please explain why.
15. Have you talked with anyone else about your decision?
    Yes ___ Who? _____
    (relationship)
    No ___

16. Does he (she) agree with you? Yes ___ No ___ Don't know ___
17. Would you like to talk over your decision with anybody?
    Yes ___ Who? (check)
    doctor ___ nurse ___ friend ___ clergyman ___ social worker ___ family ___ other ___
    No ___

185

186

18. a. Before this pregnancy were you using any birth control? Yes ___
    No ___
    b. Were you using birth control at the time you became pregnant?
    Yes ___ No ___

19. If yes, which one(s)?
    Pill ___
    Loop/coil/IUD ___
    Condom/safe ___
    Diaphragm ___
    Foam ___
    Rhythm ___
    Douche ___
    Withdrawal ___
    Other (specify) ___

20. If no, why haven't you used birth control? Please check which reasons below.

	Generally	This time
Wanted to get pregnant	___	___
Forgot to use	___	___
Not easily available	___	___
Too expensive	___	___
Didn't think I'd get pregnant	___	___
I didn't like the idea	___	___
He didn't like the idea	___	___
Didn't have enough information	___	___
Couldn't get it without parents' approval	___	___
Afraid of what it might do to my body	___	___
Religious reasons	___	___
Other	___	___

21. After this pregnancy do you want birth control?
    Yes ___ No ___
    Pill ___
    Loop/coil/IUD ___
    Condom/safe ___
    Diaphragm ___
    Foam ___
    Rhythm ___
    Other (specify) ___
    No more children (tubes tied, sterilization) ___
    Need more information ___

_____   _____
(Date)   (Please sign your name)

Index